William Alonso Gutiérrez Sandí
Hannah Diermissen Rodríguez

NOTES ON MARITIME MEDICINE

William Alonso Gutiérrez Sandí
Hannah Diermissen Rodríguez

NOTES ON MARITIME MEDICINE

ScienciaScripts

This book is a translation from the original published under ISBN 978-620-2-11153-9.

Publisher:
Sciencia Scripts
is a trademark of
Dodo Books Indian Ocean Ltd. and OmniScriptum S.R.L publishing group

120 High Road, East Finchley, London, N2 9ED, United Kingdom
Str. Armeneasca 28/1, office 1, Chisinau MD-2012, Republic of Moldova, Europe
Printed at: see last page
ISBN: 978-620-5-71339-6

INDEX GENERAL

Dedication William Alonso Gutiérrez Sandí

To God for giving me the strength and wisdom to face this challenge, in you I can do all things, Lord.

To my father and mother for giving me the opportunity to be born, live and grow up to become a good person; as well as the emotional and economic support in the final stage of this study project. Thank you very much, mum and dad.

To Yorleni for always being there in good times and bad, for always supporting me unconditionally to move forward with all the goals I have set for myself, for being part of my life and professional projects.
Thank you my love.

To my godmother Celia Rosa, who has been unconditionally present in this new professional stage and, thanks to her support, I was able to have the opportunity to close life cycles in order to start others that have helped me to recover much of the time that had been taken away from me. Thank you very much godmother for supporting me to be reborn as the phoenix.

Dedication Hannah Diermissen Rodríguez

To the Eternal Heavenly Father for giving me life, family, vision, work, wisdom, strength and love for my profession and for the people of the coasts, especially my beloved Puerto Puntarenas, which inclined me to see their needs and to grasp the opportunities for their development.

To my children for being the engine that moves my existence, for accompanying me in my journey through life, in my struggles and challenges, I love you children, always in my heart.

To my parents for being exactly the way they are, for teaching me not to give up and to follow my dreams.

To my colleagues and friends for showing me the way and supporting me, only in this way was it possible to achieve each step of the construction of this speciality and of this final graduation work, teamwork and unity is strength.

About the Authors
William Alonso Gutierrez Sandí

William Gutierrez Sandí is a student of Medicine and Surgery at the Universidad Internacional de las Americas (UIA), Costa Rica. He holds a university specialist diploma in knowledge management from the University of Leon, Spain (2006 - 2007).

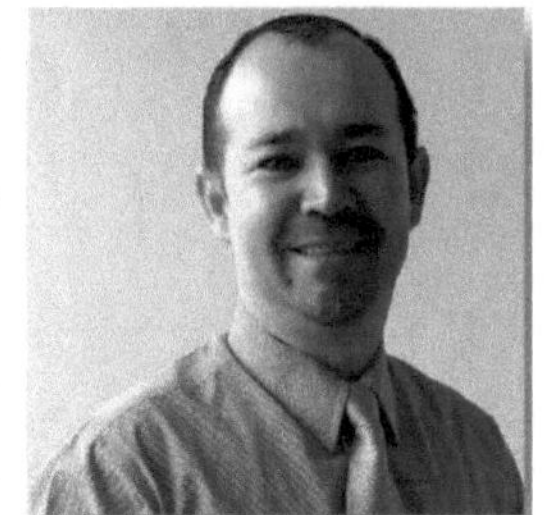

He also holds the title of Academic Doctorate in Projects, issued by the Universidad Iberoamericana Internacional (UNINI) Puerto Rico, United States (2012-2016) and his area of expertise is the management of innovation and technology projects. He completed with mention of excellent the advanced studies program for the PhD in Project Engineering at the Polytechnic University of Catalonia, Spain (2006 - 2010). Graduated with honours from the Master's programme in Project Management at the University for International Cooperation (2003 - 2004), studies with GAC certification as UCI is an authorized centre and complies with the training standards of the Project Management Institute (PMI). Graduated with mention of recognition from the bachelor's degree programme in electronic engineering at the Institute Tecnologico de Costa Rica (1996-2000).

EXPERIENCE: William A. Gutierrez Sandi has more than 15 years of experience in activities related to engineering, bioengineering and in the last 4 years has ventured into research topics related to the medical area. In addition, he has vast experience in the management of high technology projects and university teaching at undergraduate and postgraduate level, both in Costa Rica and internationally.

OTHER ACTIVITIES: William loves science, sports, especially extreme sports, biomedicine, cooking, nature and is a rescuer of animals that have been abandoned or hurt by their previous owners.

Hannah Diermissen Rodríguez

Hannah Diermissen Rodríguez holds a degree in Medicine and Surgery from the International University of the Americas (UIA), Costa Rica (1992-1997). She is a specialist in Health Services Administration with emphasis in Management from the Universidad Estatal a Distancia (UNED), Costa Rica (2002- 2006). She holds a Master's degree in Health Management (2001 2002), and also a Master's degree in Management in Development Projects (2016-2018), both from the Central American University of Public Administration (ICAP).

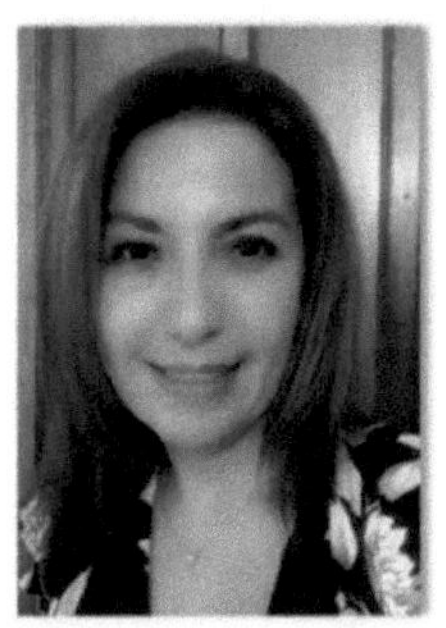

EXPERIENCE Hannah Diermissen Rodnguez has more than 20 years of experience in health centre management. She is the medical director of the health area San Rafael de Puntarenas. She is part of the Technical Coordination of Cancer in the Costa Rican Social Security Fund (CCSS), she holds the position of National Coordinator of the Oncological Rehabilitation Project. She also has experience in activities related to training and training in health management, as well as issues related to cardiac and oncological rehabilitation. In addition, she has experience in project management in areas such as health, teaching, research and social development.

OTHERS ACTIVITIES: Hannah is a keen advocate of medical science, research, social projects, support for vulnerable groups*, health of people working at sea, maritime medicine, rehabilitation, protection of the seas, animals and nature in general. Her greatest

passion is to be a mother to her beloved children.

SUMMARY

The practice of maritime medicine requires the professional to have a series of aptitudes and competencies that include in-depth knowledge of the subject, professional ethics, written and oral communication skills, the ability to work in teams and interact with professionals from different areas, handling multidisciplinary issues, an openness to deal with multiculturalism, and knowledge of medical administration to propose, lead and manage projects that involve relations with public, private and academic actors and international organisations to meet the requirements for the transport of people and goods at the international level.

Training in maritime medicine is not traditionally covered as such during the undergraduate degree in medicine and surgery in many medical schools internationally. However, the University of Cadiz has a separate postgraduate course dedicated exclusively to the subject, which is of great value to medical professionals with the necessary knowledge to practice in this professional area at an international level.

Maritime medical personnel are responsible for the prevention, inspection and treatment of acute and chronic pathologies related to maritime occupational medicine and commercial, sporting, recreational, etc. activities related to the relationship between human beings and the aquatic environment. During the training process in this discipline, the different medical professionals who wish to acquire more specific knowledge, as well as medical skills and knowledge about seafarers and companies, will be trained in subjects related to the history and fundamentals of maritime medicine, about the requirements to perform medical examinations and international regulations applied in maritime medicine, as well as different common pathologies that are related to the activities of seafarers.

By definition, maritime activities are dangerous; work on ships, docks, sports and other activities carried out by seafarers is dangerous. Therefore, as part of the training activities in the speciality programme in maritime medicine, the study of regulations related to occupational risk prevention, safety, regulations and emergencies applied to medicine in the maritime field was carried out, as well as topics related to underwater medicine activities such as: the principles of physiology, criteria, requirements in the assessment of fitness in diving and some pathologies of emergencies in the maritime field. In addition, the reader is provided with some quick bibliographical references on pathologies, principles of accident management, rescue and first aid in aquatic environments that are part of the healthcare activity that doctors specialising in the care of patients who practise sports and/or aquatic activities must carry out.

Therefore, it is in the author's interest in representing this book that it should enable future students entering formal study in maritime medicine to have a notion of what the exit activities will be, the knowledge they will be able to acquire through the readings they will find in this compendium, as well as the professional sub-areas in which they will be able to work so that they can give the appropriate value to this medical speciality.

INTRODUCTION

Maritime medicine represents an area of medicine that has origins dating back to Egyptian, Greek, Roman, Viking and European times. Seafarers have been the pioneers in the exploration of new continents, they have accessed territories that have given humanity access to resources found in other regions and which must be moved to be enjoyed, industrialised and consumed by people. This not only allows the improvement of living conditions, but also of the health of populations, the transport of goods that helps the development of the global economy. However, even though the application of medicine, public health and occupational medicine has always been related to the subject of seafarers and seafarers, it is only at the end of the 20th century that it began to be formalised as a specialised discipline in the medical field, which claims an important place in the fields of medical specialities.

At international level there are national maritime authorities such as: Danish Maritime Authority, Dutch Maritime Authority, Finnish Maritime Administration, German Maritime Authority, Hong Kong Marine Department, Icelandic Maritime Administration, Malta Maritime Authority, Norwegian Maritime Directorate, Swedish Maritime Administration, UK Maritime and Coastguard Agency, US Maritime Authority, as well as national maritime health associations mentioned above which regulate maritime health activities according to the ordinances of the Ministries of Health and different public and private actors in each country. The above-mentioned national maritime health associations regulate the health activity in accordance with the ordinances of the Ministries of Health and different public and private actors in each country.

For this reason, there is a need in most Latin American countries to promote the training of professionals in this discipline, the teaching of which is not very well developed in medical degree curricula. Seafaring professionals and workers must have a series of knowledge and notions in the field of medicine, in order to know how to act and respond to certain health complications that may arise in their day-to-day work, in a working environment where medical care is complex.

During the training of the specialist in maritime medicine at the University of Cadiz, the aim is for the student to develop adequate training to specialise in the field of health care in maritime environments, taking into account the special considerations and particularities that occur in them, developing the knowledge of maritime medicine, passing through the study of maritime medicine in sport or aquatic and hyperbaric medicine, as well as occupational safety and occupational medicine in the maritime field. Many of these training activities require the creation of academic activity reports, which have been integrated into this book, and can be used by other healthcare professionals as a bibliographic reference, so that they can have an idea of what professional activities they will be exposed to in the future as a doctor specialising in maritime medicine.

There are currently academic centres at international level which are affiliated to IMHA that conduct research and postgraduate training in maritime medicine, e.g. IMHA's Maritime Medicine Research Unit, the University of Costa Rica, the

International Seafarers' Research Centre, L'UBO, the University of Western Brittany, the World Maritime University, as well as education, outreach and open training programmes in maritime medicine by IMHA's member associations in different countries.

The speciality of maritime medicine is a different and separate medical speciality within traditional medicine, due to its inherent connotations, which integrates multidisciplinary knowledge such as occupational medicine, emergencies, occupational safety, telemedicine, internal medicine, applied to aquatic and maritime environments and therefore may denote that seafarers are people with different needs in their management with respect to the management of the traditional patient.

Let us enter this ocean of knowledge, let the rivers of knowledge carry our illusions and expectations so that at the end of the road, we can count on the peace of an autumn sunset in front of a lake with its calm waters, because we can have the knowledge that will improve the lives of these seafarers.

Let us remember that the sea always provides each person with what he or she needs to survive.

CHAPTER I. HISTORY AND FUNDAMENTALS OF MARITIME MEDICINE

History of Medicine. The age of rowing.

Author: Hannah Diermissen Rodríguez
Email: hannahdiermissen@gmail.com

The part on naval history was very interesting because, as we commented, the history of navigation throughout the centuries is unquestionably linked to the appearance and subsequent resolution, in most cases, of multiple health problems that arose due to the fact that man found himself in a hostile environment such as the sea, where the isolated sailor on a ship with multiple hygienic deficiencies had to find his own way to survive.

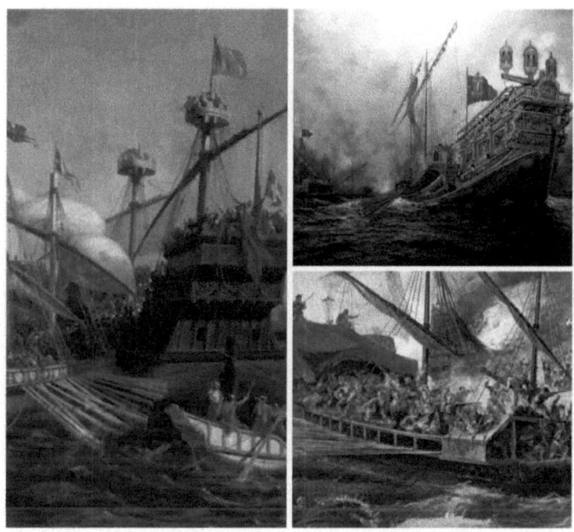

Figure 01. Slavery in the Spanish galleys of the 18th century.
Source: https://revistadehistoria.es/la-esclavitud-en-las-galeras-espanolas-del-siglo-xviii/

Dr. Canals (2012) in an article available on the website el medico interactivo mentions: *"Maritime Medicine, a discipline with anchors in the past, active in the present and with prospects for the future. In Maritime Medicine, the subject of concern in terms of health is the person who is in close contact with the water or the sea, let us call him or her a sailor, diver, bather, water sportsman and, above all, the seafaring worker. In the latter case, we would be dealing with Maritime Occupational Medicine. By appealing to the internationality of the waters, we would also enter into Traveller's Medicine, which is in contact with all kinds of diseases, the spread of which via the sea has made its mark on the history of mankind, and Tropical Medicine as diseases imported from the professional sphere. If we turn our eyes to the relationship with the ship or "vessel", names such as nautical or naval come to mind: Nautical or Naval Medicine.*

The documents begin by dividing the stages of navigation into three main groups. For this purpose, the authors Schadewaldt and Goethe (1984) distinguish three periods in the history of maritime medicine:

- o The era of oar propulsion.
- o The age of sail propulsion.
- o Age of machine propulsion (steam, internal combustion and nuclear propulsion).

For the purposes of the scope of this paper, we focus on events during the rowing stage.

Navigation with oars. Sanitary conditions of crew members.

The age of oar propulsion is considered the worst for the sanitary conditions of seafarers. The galleys (ships propelled by oarsmen known as galley slaves).

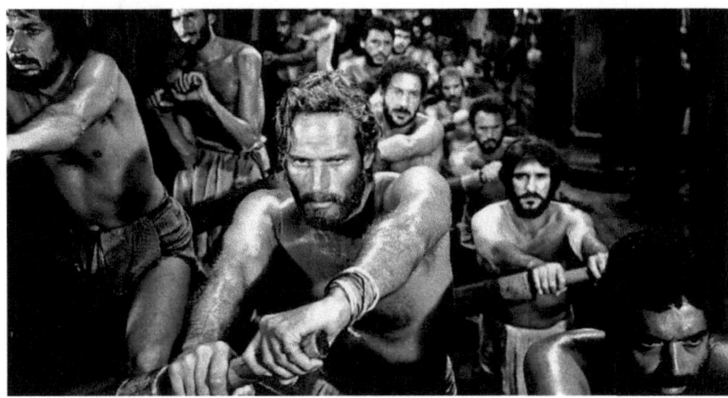

Figure 02. Depiction of slaves and prisoners in the galleys, taken from the 1959 film Ben Hur.
Source: https://hips.hearstapps.com/hmg-prod.s3.amazonaws.com/images/benhur-1538607909.png

Phoenicians, Carthaginians, Athenians, Romans, none of them had well-established codes for the regulation of sanitary standards in the galleys run by slaves or criminals who were not sentenced for more than 10 years because sending them to the galley was tantamount to a death sentence.

The Spartans are the ones who, according to Garrison (1921), apparently later had military doctors on board their ships. Therefore, we can safely say that the galleys had the worst hygienic and sanitary conditions in the history of navigation; on these ships, the galley slave (oarsman) was the main driving force; and as mentioned above, this work was carried out almost exclusively by slaves, prisoners of war or those condemned to the galleys.

Fortunately for the crew and sailors, as they progress through the stages of navigation, health conditions improve, because in ancient times on civilian ships, rowers were considered to be replaceable and on military ships, the focus was on the total destruction of the other fleet, with no thought for the crew.

An important historical event in this period was the era of rowing, which was an important historical event.

Bibliographical references.

1. Canals, M. (2012). Maritime Medicine, a discipline anchored in the past, active in the present and with prospects for the future. El medico interactivo. [Accessed 21 Sep 2021]. Available at: https://elmedicointeractivo.com/medicina-maritima-disciplina-anclajes-pasado-activa-presente-y-perspectivas-futuro-20121017111138075445/

2. GARRISON, H. (1921). History of Medicine. Espasa-Calpe. Madrid, Spain.

3. SCHADEWALDT, H. and GOETHE, W.H.G. (1984). The History of Nautical Medicine. In Goethe, W.H.G.; Watson, E. and Jones,E. (eds.): "Handbook of Nautical Medicine". Springer-Verlag. Berlin, pp.3-19.

Standards and regulations in maritime medicine. International Convention on Standards of Training, Certification and Watchkeeping for Seafarers (STCW).

Author: William Gutiérrez Sandí
Email: wgutierrezs@hotmail.com

As can be seen from the readings provided, the conventions are the pillars of maritime law. They suggest how to design national maritime laws to ensure compatibility across national jurisdictions or to standardise national maritime laws (IMO, 2009).

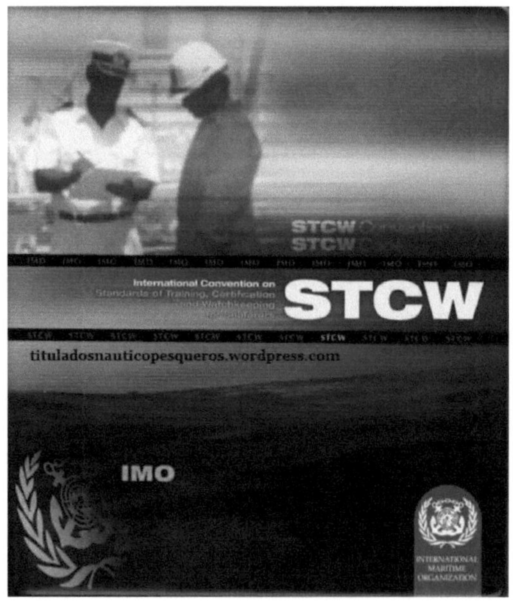

Figure 03. The STCW GUIDE FOR SEAFARERS. Contains the 2010 Manila amendments.
Source: https://tituladosnauticopesqueros.files.wordpress.com/2017/02/stcw1.jpg

As Antoni Fernández Parera referred in 2010 to Siri Pettersen Strandenes' document on international maritime conventions and regulations, in 2009, the IMO had 169 member states and three associate members. It works through committees: the Maritime Safety Committee, the Environment and Security Committee, the Technical Cooperation Committee, the Legal Committee and the Facilitation Committee. There are several subcommittees, one of which is the national flag implementation subcommittee under the maritime safety committee, which works on the implementation of the conventions.

- o The International Convention S.T.C.W74/95/10 and (For Fisheries STCW-F/95) together with two other International Maritime Bureau Conventions, the S.O.L.A.S and MAR.POL. is one of the four pillars of the international regulatory regime for shipping and maritime fisheries.

- o The Convention on Training and Certification of Fishing Vessel Personnel (STCW-F/95) will enter into force on 29 September 2012, having reached the required 15 ratifications. Good news for our colleagues working in this sector.

- o BOE of the provision: https://www.boe.es/buscar/doc.php?id=BOE-A-2012-3748.

The site Titulad@s Náutico Pesqueros indicates in an article of 25 February 2017:

"In June 2010, a diplomatic conference in Manila adopted a comprehensive and far-reaching set of amendments to the International Convention on Standards of Training, Certification and Watchkeeping for Seafarers, 1978, popularly known as the STCW Convention, and its associated Code. This instrument is considered one of the four pillars of the international regulatory regime for shipping, along with two other IMO Conventions: SOLAS and MARPOL, and the ILO Maritime Labour Convention. The amendments adopted mark the first major revision of the instrument since those adopted in 1995, which completely revised the 1978 STCW Convention. The shipping industry depends on competent and well-trained seafarers to ensure safety of life at sea, maritime security, efficiency of navigation and the protection and preservation of the marine environment. The objective of the STCW Convention as amended is to establish the international standards necessary for training establishments and educators to develop the skills and competencies required of today's seafarers. The ITF prepared this guide to help seafarers understand the revisions and locate the information of most interest to them. I support this effort to ensure that the requirements of the Convention are accessible to all seafarers and hope that this guide will help to meet the objectives of the STCW Convention and Code.

Koji Sekimizu Secretary-General, IMO".

These operational and regulatory steps are in direct line of action with the operational scheme in terms of how the management process for the promulgation of regulations is managed. This is a very lengthy process, involving many committees and sub-committees, and which finally has to be ratified by the governments of the countries where the ships arrive in port.

An example of the process of developing regulations and applicable articles can be found in document U.2 Regulations of the University of Cadiz (2021):

"An example of IMO (International Maritime Organisation) conventions for the case of certification and watchkeeping of

seafarers in order to achieve international certification (also includes regulations related to medical examinations, e.g. minimum visual acuity according to professional category): "International Convention on Standards of Training, Certification and Watchkeeping for Seafarers (STCW)", 1978; the Convention was adopted on 7-7-78, was internationally applicable as of 28-4-84, was amended or corrected in 1995 with international application as of 1-2-97 [Enter IMO, STCW] and the last update are the so-called Manila Amendments or Manila Convention in 2010. Most of the countries that have signed up to it are still in the process of applying for such certification, they form the "White list" [document in pdf, as of 5-6-03], in Uk and other countries serve as a basis for accepting international certificates".

A good example of a matter that STCW regulates is in relation to the vision of crew members, which is included in the white list of international regulations.

On this point, it may be noted that the main instruments used by the STWC for the medical examination of seafarers are as follows:

World Labour Organisation (UNWTO).
   o The Medical Examination of Young Persons (Sea) Convention, 1921 (n. 16).

   o The Convention on the Medical Examination of Seafarers. 1946 (n.73).

   o The Convention on the Protection of Health and Medical Care (marines) 1987 (n.164).

   o The recommendation on medical advice at sea, 1958 (n.106).

   o The UNWTO Convention on Occupational Health Services 1985 (n.161).

   o The recommendation (n.171) and the ethical technical guidelines for workers' health surveillance (1997).

International Maritime Organisation (IMO, IMO).
The STCW Convention, 1978, as amended in 1995.

World Health Organisation (WHO).
WHO resolutions WHA 14.51:
   o EB 29.R10.

   o WHA 15.21.

   o EB 37.R25.

   o EB 43.R23.

These documents can be validated from the source: http://www.ilo.org/public/english/dialoguesector/techmeet/ilowho97/meden2.htm #Heading4.

Another example is the tripartite cooperation between IMO, UNWTO and WHO on guidelines for the conduct of regular and pre-sea medical examinations of seafarers (1997).

Bibliographical references.

1. Fernández, A. (2012). Translation of the Textbook of Maritime Medicine - Manual of Maritime Medicine. Siri Pettersen Strandenes. Plataforma e-learnig FUECA-UCA . [Accessed 22 Sep 2021]. Available at: https://av02-ext.uca.es/moodle/course/view.php?id=4256

2. IMO (2009). Conventions, International Maritime Organisation, London. [Accessed 22 Sep 2021]. Available at: https://www.imo.org/en/About/Conventions/Pages/ListOfConventions.aspx

3. Nautical fishing certificates. International legislation, national legislation and STCW guidance for seafarers. Contains the 2010 Manila amendments. [Accessed 22 Sep 2021]. Available at: https://tituladosnauticopesqueros.wordpress.com/2017/02/25/guia-stcw-para-la-gente-de-mar-contiene-las-enmiendas-de-manila-2010-stcw95-uno-de-los-cuatro-pilares-del-regimen-regulatorio-internacional-del-transporte-maritimo-junto-con-otros-dos-convenios-omi/

4. University of Cadiz. U2. Regulations. FUECA-UCA e-learning platform. [Accessed 22 Set 2021]. Available at: https://av02-ext.uca.es/moodle/course/view.php?id=4256

CHAPTER II. MEDICAL EXAMINATIONS AND INTERNATIONAL STANDARDS APPLIED IN MARITIME MEDICINE

Maritime Health Management / Organización de la Medicina Marítima / Maritime Health Management. Current situation in Costa Rica.

Author: Hannah Diermissen Rodríguez
Email: hannahdiermissen@gmail.com

In Costa Rica, maritime medicine is unknown to a large part of the medical profession. In fact, medical curricula do not include any subject on the subject. Moreover, no medical examination certificates are issued for seafarers. This coming Sunday there will be elections in Costa Rica, and one of the candidates includes in his proposals that he will promote the inclusion of Maritime Medicine and Maritime Nursing and promote the issuance of the "Medical Certificate for Services at Sea". In other words, information about this branch of medicine is already reaching the media.

With regard to training for other professions, as of 1 December 2014, the National Institute of Apprenticeship has been offering the Basic Embarkation Course, which is compulsory for crew members of national vessels. Without this approved course, it is not possible to sail. Due to the pandemic, a refresher course for the Basic Embarkation Course will be held from 2020 onwards. The current global situation has optimised the study facilities. Although some activities require face-to-face attendance, such as sea training, many academic activities can be done remotely, which is a relief for people who find It Inconvenient to miss work and travel several days to other cities. For example, a group of medical colleagues will soon be doing this course on the Pacific coast of the country, and among them there are two who live in the Atlantic area. The asynchronous virtuality of the theoretical part of the course means that they can continue with their daily work and that the financial outlay is not necessary.

In short, in my country, seafarer-related training is gaining ground and positioning itself in the official landscape, which I believe is necessary to be able to provide a better service to the population involved in aquatic affairs.

Bibliographical references.

1. Guanacaste at altitude. [Internet]. [Accessed 3 Feb 2022]. Available at https://www.guanacastealaaltura.com/index.php/el-pais/item/1411-ina-capacita-a-tripulantes-de-embarcaciones

2. National Learning Institute. [Internet]. [Accessed 3 Feb 2022]. Available from
https://www.ina.ac.cr/Noticias/Lists/EntradasDeBlog/Post.aspx?ID=68

3. President Figueres. [Internet]. [Accessed 3 Feb 2022]. Available at https://www.presidentefigueres.cr/

Case studies on medical fitness for seafarers' medical certificates.

Case I. Patient with ETS. Assessment for the seafarer's medical certificate of embarkation.

Author: William Gutiérrez Sandí
Email: wgutierrezs@hotmail.com

For this exercise we will develop the case of Danny, a young 28 year old sailor, who graduated as a naval engineer 3 years ago at the University of Costa Rica, who carried out his medical examination in Panama in 2020 and whose medical examination expires in February 2022, so he needs to renew it. Danny has been working as a bridge officer for two years.

However, our young officer has Primary Arterial Hypertension (HTA), controlled, with check-ups every six months with his family doctor, blood chemistry control tests, and complementary tests with chest x-ray, annual electrocardiogram, the above for his circulatory pathology.

In addition, every 2 years he must undergo ophthalmology tests, audiometry and functional tests to determine the proper state of the musculoskeletal system.

Danny reports HB: 14.3, Ht: 42, Platelets 325.000, WBC: 8.000, fasting glycaemia by micromethod: 88 mg/dl, Total Cholesterol: 196, C. LDL: 110, C. HDL: 56, Triglycerides: 147, EGO: no data of glucosuria, No toxic urine. Chest X-ray normal, EKG within normal parameters.

The patient's main treatments for hypertension are: enalapril 20 mg daily by mouth (angiotensin-converting enzyme inhibitors), Atenolol 50 mg daily by mouth (beta-blocker). Weekly ambulatory blood pressure monitoring (ABPM) record for the last eight weeks indicates:

Table 01. Ambulatory blood pressure monitoring record (ABPM).

Date	Systolic Blood Pressure	Diastolic Blood Pressure	Heart rate
15.12.21	116	82	63
22.12.21	126	76	71
02.01.22	131	69	76
11.01.22	105	78	74
15.01.22	114	86	86

21.01.22	112	81	89
01.02.22	119	73	91
08.02.22	124	84	67

Source: Patient data under study by Ambulatory Blood Pressure Monitoring (ABPM).

Therefore, the patient with the medication he uses, the radiographic, electrocardiac, biochemical, haematological tests carried out, we observe that he satisfies the requirements established in the BOE 313. 31.12.2007, in relation to the Guidelines for carrying out medical examinations of seafarers. WCMS 2017, STCW GUIDE FOR SEAFARERS. FITT (ITF) and the criteria for the management of adult patients with cardiac pathology established by the Costa Rican Social Security Fund (Caja Costarricense del Seguro Social); the aforementioned based on the following items.

Guidelines for the conduct of medical examinations of seafarers / International Labour Office, Sectoral Activities Programme; International Maritime Organization. - Geneva: ILO, 2013, in Part 3. Guidance for persons authorized by competent authorities to conduct medical examinations and issue medical certificates X. The importance of medical examination for safety and health on board ship: "The medical practitioner should be aware of the importance of medical examination for the promotion of safety and health at sea and for the assessment of the fitness of seafarers to perform routine and emergency duties and to live on board...", "... Medication for the medical examination should be administered by the medical practitioner...". ... Seafarers' medication should be carefully evaluated as it may cause disqualification due to side effects that cannot be easily managed at sea. Where a medicine is essential to control a life-threatening condition, the inability to take it could have serious consequences". It is therefore correct that the assessing physician should be aware of the appropriate primary care or primary medical management of the naval officer in order that he or she may be considered fit to embark and that the medical condition does not present a problem on board.

The Guidelines for the Conduct of Medical Fitness Examinations for Seafarers, Annex C, Fitness Requirements, indicates that fitness requirements for work at sea vary considerably and should cover both routine and emergency tasks. Functions that may require assessment include: endurance; stamina; energy; flexibility; balance and coordination; size: adequate to enter confined spaces; capacity for physical activity: heart and respiratory rates; and fitness to perform specific tasks: use of a breathing apparatus. Table B-I/9 provides recommendations on the physical fitness to be assessed for seafarers whose work is governed by the STCW, 1978, as amended, based on the tasks performed at sea, in this case our patient complies with them.

However, it is in Annex D, Criteria relating to medical fitness for medication purposes, that the regulation and care to be taken by the assessing physician in this respect is indicated: "*The examining physician shall assess the known adverse effects of all medications used and the reaction they cause in the individual. The use of a specific medication for certain conditions listed in Annex*

E is noted in relation to that condition. Where medication is clinically essential for the effective management of a condition, e.g. insulin, anticoagulants and medication for mental health conditions, it is dangerous to discontinue it in order to be fit for work at sea. The physician should be very conscious of the need for the seafarer to have documentation for the use of his or her medication.

For the case of Danny our patient under study and according to what is indicated in Annex E it is considered that:

- o With regard to the guidelines for the conduct of medical examinations of seafarers, WCMS 2017, in Annex E. Criteria relating to physical fitness, with respect to common conditions, and in accordance with ICD-10 classification criteria, diagnostic codes, I00-99 Cardiovascular system, Hypertension Increased likelihood of ischaemic heart disease, eye and liver damage and stroke. Possibility of an acute hypertensive episode.

    - o Incompatible with the reliable performance of routine and emergency tasks in a Safe and effective manner. expected to be temporary (T), expected to be permanent (P).

        - T - usually if systolic pressure >160 or diastolic pressure >100 mmHg until investigated and treated according to national or international guidelines for the management of hypertension.

        - P - with a systolic pressure >160 or diastolic pressure >100 mmHg persistent with or without treatment.

    - o Able to perform some but not all tasks or to work in some but not all waters (R). More frequent supervision is needed (L).

        - L - if additional monitoring is necessary to ensure that the level remains within national guidelines.

    - o Able to perform all tasks anywhere in the world in the assigned section.

        - If treated according to national guidelines and there are no disabling effects from the condition or medication.

    Given that the patient presents stable BP values, with stable treatment for the last 24 months, with good adherence to treatment, with no acute episodes in the last months, this condition would not be a criterion for the non-issuance of the medical certificate.

In relation to the issue of migraine, the royal decree of the BOE 313.31.12.2007 indicates ANNEX II, Criteria for the assessment of fitness for embarkation, 2.9. Diseases of the circulatory system. For the purpose of assessing fitness, the following criteria shall always be taken into account: family history of heart disease or sudden death, presence of symptoms and/or signs, functional capacity, location, prognosis, presence of electrocardiographic and/or echocardiographic abnormalities suggesting severe cardiac pathology even in the absence of symptoms, possibilities of treatment on board, risk of severe symptoms on board, risk factors and/or associated complications, therapy involving restrictions or limitations for the normal performance of their activities and specialist report. 2.9.1.7 Essential hypertension with significant organic repercussions or hypertension.

Regarding the follow-up criteria for chronic patients with HTN management by the CCSS in Costa Rica, patients must have blood pressures SBP less than 140 mmHg and DBP less than 90 mmHg in their 6-monthly controls, as well as lipid values within the parameters of the American Heart Association.

Therefore, in summary, our patient meets the criteria of international guidelines for the embarkation of marine officers, as well as the criteria used by the CCSS for the management of the chronic patient with controlled arterial hypertension, with medication that does not involve the use of authorisations because it is controlled medication. For the purposes of this case, it is an example of a chronic, controlled patient who can embark, carry out his professional activity without endangering his life or the health of other crew members under regular conditions.

Bibliographical references.

1. Guidelines for the conduct of medical examinations of seafarers. [Internet]. [Accessed 9 Feb 2022]. Available from https://www.ilo.org/wcmsp5/groups/public/---ed_dialogue/---sector/documents/normativeinstrument/wcms_174796.pdf

2. STCW Guide for Seafarers. ITGLWF. [Internet]. [Accessed 9 Feb 2022]. Available from https://www.itfglobal.org/es/reports-publications/guia-stcw-para-la-gente-de-mar

3. Guidelines for the detection, diagnosis and treatment of arterial hypertension in the Caja Costarricense del Seguro Social. [Internet]. [Accessed 3 Feb 2022]. Available at https://www.binasss.sa.cr/protocolos/hipertension.pdf

4. Royal Decree 1696/2007 of 14 December 2007, regulating medical examinations for maritime embarkation. [Internet]. [Accessed 3 Feb 2022]. Available at https://www.boe.es/eli/es/rd/2007/12/14/1696

Case II. Comparison of medical examination systems with ILO/IMO parameters. Medical examinations. Neurological system.

Author: William Gutiérrez Sandí
Email: wgutierrezs@hotmail.com

A review of the literature shows that the 2010 STCW Seafarers' Guide. FITT 2010 makes reference to the health care of officers and seafarers, following the 2010 amendment of the original 1973 document. However, it makes no specific mention of the care to be taken for seafarers with underlying nervous system pathology. The Republic of the Philippines, through Administrative Order No 2007-0025 Revised Guidlines for conducting medical fitness examinations for seafarers, indicates the requirements for the Pre-Employment Medical Examination (PEME), the Pre-Licensure Examinees, as well as for the Restricted Service Health Certificate, which indicate whether there are limitations on the issuance of health certificates for seafarers. The tool differentiates between first-time seafarers and seafarers seeking to renew their medical certificate. In the annex entitled: Minimum Test Requirements, on page 3, it indicates the evaluation guide format, and on pages 5 - 6 it indicates the minimum requirements necessary to accredit good health for the issuance of the seafarer's certificate. In relation to the issue of central nervous system pathologies, it states as pathologies to be assessed: "*There shall be no existing manifestation of an acute or chronic neurological or sensory disorder. Careful assessment should be made of any significant past history of such conditions that may recur or limit functional ability to perform at sea and require medical attention or periodic monitoring, including but not limited to the following. Nervous System Conditions: Ataxia, active (gait instability), Impairment of central nervous system function resulting from secondary or active medical conditions, e.g., Diabetes, Toxic Reaction, and Diabetes, Toxic Reaction and Thyroid Disorder, Migraine, frequent seizures causing disability, Narcolepsy or Sleep Disorders resulting in unpredictable sleepiness when the individual is awake, Post-Concussion Syndrome, Active, Seizure Disorder Secondary to structural abnormality, epilepsy, alcohol or drugs, withdrawal or metabolic disorder, stroke, syncope and other disorders of consciousness, tremors, active, interfering with fine motor functions, vertigo, central or peripheral origin, sense organ disorders: cholesteatoma until successful surgical intervention, chronic mastoiditis of both ears, Chronic Otitis Media, Chronic Sinusitis until successful surgical intervention, Frequent Epistaxis*" to name the most frequent.

In the case of the format used in the United Kingdom, in the document GUIDELINES FOR APPROVED CLINICS, used for the UK P&I Club's Pre-Employment Medical Examination (PEME) programme, which aims to implement the standards set by the UK Maritime and Coastguard Authority (MCA) are used by all examining doctors to determine whether a seafarer is fit for sea service, however, it does not explicitly state which pathologies related to the nervous system should be assessed. However, the UK Maritime and Coastguard Agency's 2010 Approved Doctor's Manual Seafarer Medical Examinations in Chapter 7 discusses the clinical assessment of conditions such as loss of consciousness, altered consciousness, epilepsy and sleep disorders, providing assessment conditions and algorithms for clinical actions to be taken for these conditions.

In Europe, the EUROPEAN COMMITTEE FOR DRAWING UP STANDARDS IN THE FIELD OF INLAND NAVIGATION, in its 2018 edition, also indicates in the European Standard for Qualifications in Inland Navigation (ES-QIN), the following pathologies as assessable at the time of carrying out a study of the patient for the issuance of a medical certificate for boarding: "*seizures, epilepsy, migraine, sleep apnoea, syncope, narcolepsy, multiple sclerosis, Parkinson's disease, as well as neurosurgical processes*". The document adds the guidelines to be fulfilled in order to give the document as compliant or non-compliant.

On the other hand, in Spain there is the ROYAL DECREE 1696/2007, of 14 December, which regulates the medical examinations for maritime embarkation; which in ANNEX II. Criteria for the assessment of fitness for embarkation indicates which pathologies are subject to study when issuing the medical certificate for embarkation. In section 2.6 Diseases of the nervous system. For the purpose of assessing fitness, the following criteria should always be taken into account: presence of symptoms and/or signs, probability of occurrence of severe symptoms on board, therapy involving restrictions or limitations for the normal performance of their activities and a specialist's report. *2.6.1 Encephalic, spinal and peripheral nervous system diseases resulting in loss or reduction of motor, sensory or coordination functions, syncopal episodes, tremors or spasms affecting the ability to work. 2.6.2 Epilepsy. Exceptionally, those patients with a good prognosis who have not presented seizures in the last two years, with a favourable report from the specialist, may be considered fit with restrictions. In the case of bridge personnel, this period shall be extended to five years. 2.6.3 Primary or secondary convulsive crises due to the consumption of medicines, drugs or post-surgery in the last six months. Exceptionally, those persons who provide a favourable report from a specialist may be considered suitable. 2.6.4 Balance disorders. Dizziness, instability or dizziness refractory to treatment*".

However, something common among all the models presented is that they are in accordance with the Guidelines for the conduct of medical examinations of seafarers issued by the ILO in 2013, which for each pathology uses the ICD-10 classification (diagnostic codes, G00-99 Diseases of the nervous system), and makes a location of the pathology according to the condition (justification for applying the criteria), so that the following classification outputs are obtained:

1. Incompatible with reliably performing routine and emergency tasks in a safe and efficient manner
   - expected to be temporary (T)
   - is expected to be permanent (P)
2. Able to perform some but not all tasks or to work in some but not all waters (R). More frequent supervision required (L)
3. Able to perform all tasks anywhere in the world in the assigned section.

These are pathologies that must comply with the parameters for the issuance of the medical boarding certificate:

- G40-41.
  - o Single partial crisis Harmful to the ship, to others and to oneself because of crises.
  - o Epilepsy - without provoking factors (multiple partial seizures) Harmful to the vessel, to others and to oneself due to seizures.
  - o Epilepsy - caused by alcohol, medication or head injury (multiple partial seizures) Harmful to the vessel, to others and to oneself because of seizures.
- Migraine (frequent attacks with disability) Likelihood of disabling recurrences.
- G47.
  - o Sleep apnoea Fatigue and episodes of sleep while working.
  - o Narcolepsy Fatigue and episodes of sleepiness while working.
- G00-99 not indicated separately Other organic nerve diseases, e.g. multiple sclerosis, Parkinson's disease. Recurrence and progression. Limitations of muscle power, balance, coordination and mobility.
- R55
  - o Syncope and other disorders of consciousness Recurrence causing.
  - o Syncope and other disorders of consciousness Recurrence causing injury and loss of control.
- T90
  - o Intracranial surgery/injury, including treatment of vascular disorders or severe head injury with brain damage. Harmful to the vessel, others and self due to seizures.
- Impaired cognitive, sensory or motor functions.
- Recurrence or complications of the underlying condition.

Therefore, there is an international normative basis for the assessment of seafarers, officers and port personnel, which allows for the classification, typification and follow-up of pathologies.

A second element corresponds to the risk classification of the tasks performed by seafarers, be it in port, on the bridge, in the engine room, on deck, and so on for each area of maritime activities.

In the document STCW Guide for Seafarers. FITT, with the Manila 2010 agreements, classifies the requirements by job position, with the academic, professional and practical requirements that each seafarer must fulfil in their activity. For this purpose, in the document "Digitalisation, standardisation and globalisation of information. Case study on: Diabetes and Obesity in Seafarers", reference is made to criteria for risk classification of patients according to acute and/or chronic diseases.

In addition, each country has national guidelines for the management of pathology in accordance with international standards, which allows for lower levels of prevalence of chronic diseases and results in lower costs for public health systems, which ultimately end up treating patients who are decompensated seafarers.

In summary, there are different country-specific guidelines for medical certificates for embarkation for ship's crew and for port personnel. However, they all comply with the Guidelines for the Conduct of Medical Examinations for Seafarers, and this has an impact on the risk classification of each patient's pathology, which ultimately results in the condition in which the medical certificate of embarkation is issued or not issued to the patient who is ultimately a seafarer.

Bibliographical references.

1. Compilation of CESNI resolutions Meeting on 8 November 2018. ANNEXES. CESNI. [Internet]. [Accessed 10 Feb 2022]. Available from https://av03-ext.uca.es/moodle/pluginfile.php/43195/mod_resource/intro/Europe%20Inland%20Navigation%20Standards%20Medical%20Fitness%20Criteria%202018.pdf

2. Digitisation, standardisation and globalisation of information. Case study on: Diabetes and Obesity in Seafarers. [Internet]. [Accessed 9 Feb 2022]. Available at https://av03-ext.uca.es/moodle/pluginfile.php/43196/mod_url/intro/Digitalisation%2C%20Obesity.pdf

3. Guidelines for the conduct of medical examinations of seafarers. [Internet]. [Accessed 9 Feb 2022]. Available from https://www.ilo.org/wcmsp5/groups/public/---ed_dialogue/---sector/documents/normativeinstrument/wcms_174796.pdf

4. Explanatory notice for the CESNI standards for medical fitness. CESNI. [Internet]. [Accessed 10 Feb 2022]. Available at https://av03-ext.uca.es/moodle/pluginfile.php/43195/mod_resource/intro/Explanations%20on%20Inland%20Navigation%20MF%20Standards.pdf

5. STCW Guide for Seafarers. ITGLWF. [Internet]. [Accessed 9 Feb 2022]. Available from https://www.itfglobal.org/es/reports-publications/guia-stcw-para-la-gente-de-mar

6. GUIDELINES FOR APPROVED CLINICS The definitive standards for all approved clinics when part of the PEME programme. [Internet]. [Accessed 10 Feb 2022]. Available from https://av03-ext.uca.es/moodle/pluginfile.php/43195/mod_resource/intro/PEME%20Cruise%20Ships.pdf

7. MCA. Approved Doctor's Manual Seafarer Medical Examinations. January 2010. [Internet]. [Accessed 10 Feb 2022]. Available from https://av03-

ext.uca.es/moodle/pluginfile.php/43195/mod_resource/intro/Guidelines%
20MCA%2C%20UK.pdf

8. Royal Decree 1696/2007 of 14 December 2007, regulating medical examinations for maritime embarkation. [Internet]. [Accessed 3 Feb 2022]. Available at https://www.boe.es/eli/es/rd/2007/12/14/1696

9. Revised Guidlines for conducting medical fitness examinations for seafarers. [Internet]. [Accessed 10 Feb 2022]. Available from https://av03-ext.uca.es/moodle/pluginfile.php/43195/mod_resource/intro/PEME%20P hillipines.pdf

CHAPTER III. MARITIME MEDICINE

Maritime occupational hazards and accidents.

Author: Hannah Diermissen Rodríguez
Email: hannahdiermissen@gmail.com

Knowledge of terms such as: boats, leeward, cross-water, fin, etc. is important for the care of a patient (not to aggravate them in a transfer) as is familiarity with the handling of a Mayo-Hegar needle holder, for example.

Medical care at sea has a number of specific characteristics such as: having a diagnostic approach which is uncertain as it is generally carried out by radio according to the skipper's impressions. The initial therapeutic approach is delegated to a non-health professional and depends on his or her health training and the suitability of the ship's first aid kit and medical equipment.

Direct action on the patient by health personnel is not immediate, and one of the fundamental differences with hospital facilities is that the environmental conditions are not, in general, ideal for the treatment of the sick or injured.

The transfer of the patient from his or her ship to a hospital ship or a hospital on land does not usually require the intervention of the medical team. This transfer is carried out with the exclusive help of the crew of the boats or fast rescue boats (FRB). These boats are usually operated by paramedics who, with sufficient experience, can handle these uncomplicated cases.

In some cases, the patient does not have sufficient autonomy for the medical staff to carry out the appropriate manoeuvres from a technical point of view. Initial stabilisation and mobilisation, even in their own boat, is the responsibility of the care team.

Paramedic rescuers and members of the patient's boat crew can provide valuable assistance in these serious cases, if they are properly organised and coordinated. However, this requires the availability of equipment such as speedboats and rescue boats, which are vessels similar to conventional inflatable boats (zodiac type), but with technical specifications defined in regulations. Their requirements are set out in IMO MSC/Circular 809/4.1: "Recommendations for reversible liferafts, self-righting liferafts and fast rescue boats, including tests, for ro-ro ferries and passenger ships".

However, things do not always go well and it is necessary to have protocols for risk management, accidents or abandonment of the boat. To this end, medical personnel and crew should be instructed in the use of the raft and supervision of their emergency crews, should avoid immersion if possible (hypothermia-ventricular fibrillation), a very important element is to avoid sudden immersion, as well as to use immersion suits or, at least, a significant amount of warm clothing (preferably wool), use buoyancy devices and take anti-Kinetosis medication before boarding the raft if the patient or crew member presents hyperemesis.

Bibliographical references.

1. http://www.cirm.it : International Medical Radio Centre of Rome (Italy)

2. http://www.sasemar.es/index.html : Sociedad de Salvamento Marítimo (Maritime Rescue Society)

3. http://www.semm.org : Spanish Society of Maritime Medicine

4. http://www.who.int/home-page : World Health Organisation

5. International Maritime Organisation (IMO) : International Maritime Organisation

6. O.I.T.: Health protection and medical care for seafarers. International Labour Conference 74th Maritime Session. Report IV. Geneva, 1987.

7. PIEDROLA GIL, G. and PIEDROLA ANGULO, G.: Medicina Preventiva Naval. In Piédrola Gil, G.: "Medicina Preventiva y Social: Higiene y Sanidad Ambiental". Ed. Amaro. Madrid, 1982, T.II, pp.: 492 and ff.

8. Royal Decree 39/97 of 17 January, approving the Prevention Services Regulations.

Marine medicine. Regulatory framework for the assessment of seafarers and associated musculoskeletal pathologies.

Author: William Gutiérrez Sandí
Email: wgutierrezs@hotmail.com

The pathologies suffered by seafarers are very diverse: infectious, digestive, traumatic, osteoarticular, osteotendinous, and the most complicated part is that they usually occur. An interesting review of the Spanish regulations applicable to the assessment of patients who may present musculoskeletal disorders due to handling loads. From a legal perspective, Law 14/1986 of 25 April 1986 on General Health establishes that the Public Administrations will develop, among others, actions for the protection, promotion and improvement of Occupational Health. Law 31/1.995 of 8 November 1995 on the Prevention of Occupational Risks, and specifically article 6 of the same, foresees that regulations must establish and specify the more technical elements of the preventive measures.

Royal Decree 487/1997 of 14 April 1997 on Minimum Health and Safety Provisions for the Manual Handling of Loads involving risks, in particular dorsolumbar risks, for workers, specifies the minimum safety conditions for the manual handling of loads and transposes into Spanish law the content of Community Directive 90/269/EEC of 29 May. Royal Decree 487/1997 of 14 April 1997 repeals the provision of the Ministry of Labour of 15 November 1935 and the Ministerial Order of 2 June 1961 on the prohibition of arm loads exceeding 80 kilograms. However, nothing is said about the Decree of 26 July 1957 approving the Regulation on work forbidden to women and minors as dangerous and unhealthy, on the understanding that it is in force as far as minors under 18 years of age are concerned.

In the specific field of the maritime-fishing sector, different regulations have been aimed at protecting the health of seafarers. In this context, the Presidential Order of 1 March 1973, which contemplates the principles of the International Labour Organisation's conventions 16 (on medical examination of minors), 73 (on medical examination of seafarers) and 113 (on medical examination of fishermen), Royal Decree 1.414/1.981 of 3 July, on the restructuring of the Social Marine Institute, in article 2, section 5, reaffirmed in the Sixth Additional Provision of Royal Decree 39/97 of 17 January, approving the Prevention Services Regulations, Royal Decrees 285/2.002 of 22 March and 525/2.002 of 14 June, which incorporate Directive 1.99/63/CE on the organisation of seafarers' working time into Spanish law, as well as the recommendations of the World Health Organisation (WHO) for the performance of periodic and pre-embarkation medical examinations.

Also when reviewing the provisions of Royal Decree 1696/2007, of 14 December, which regulates medical examinations for maritime embarkation, Article 6, point

2, refers to the specific health protocols or not determined by the Social Marine Institute, with the aim of carrying out Health Surveillance of seafarers.

Therefore, if we take the aforementioned regulations and focus them on the assessment of musculoskeletal disorders caused by manual handling of loads, they can occur in any type of work. However, the maritime fishing sector, and more specifically the maritime fishing sector, is among the industries with the highest risk; statistics show that in Spain between 20 and 30% of the causes of permanent disability granted to maritime workers are due to diseases of the musculoskeletal system and connective tissue.

Therefore, the application of the indicated regulations at the time of patient assessment is of utmost importance in order to maintain a balance between a good quality of life for seafarers, companies, insurers and the health sector; especially as it was indicated that in Spain manual handling of loads is annually and on average the origin of approximately 22% of the registered accidents with sick leave.

Bibliographical references.

1. Order of the Presidency of 1 March 1973.

2. International Labour Organisation Convention No. 16 (Medical Examination of Young Persons).

3. International Labour Organisation Convention No. 73 (Medical Examination of Seafarers).

4. International Labour Organisation Convention No. 113 (Medical Examination of Fishermen).

5. Specific Health Surveillance Protocols. Manual Handling of Loads. Ministry of Health and Consumer Affairs.

6. Royal Decree 1696/2007, of 14 December, which regulates medical examinations for maritime embarkation.

7. Law 14/1986 of 25 April 1986 on General Health.

8. Law 31/1.995 of 8 November 1995 on the Prevention of Occupational Risks.

Organisation of maritime medicine. Seafarers' pathologies.

Author: William Gutiérrez Sandí
Email: wgutierrezs@hotmail.com

The maritime fishing sector, and more specifically the maritime fishing sector, is among the highest risk industries; statistics show that in Spain between 20-30% of the causes of permanent disability granted to maritime workers are due to diseases of the musculoskeletal system, in Spain manual handling of loads is annually and on average the origin of approximately 22% of the registered accidents with sick leave. Therefore, the application of the indicated regulations at the time of assessment of patients with injuries of the musculoskeletal system is of utmost importance.

In Spain, the issue of lumbago in seafarers is so common that there is a Royal Decree 487/1.997 of 14 April on Minimum Health and Safety Provisions relating to the Manual Handling of Loads involving risks, in particular dorsolumbar risks, for workers, which is applied together with Royal Decree 1.696/2.007, of 14 December, which regulates Medical Examinations for maritime embarkation.

The latter Royal Decree defines two types of examination: firstly, the initial medical examination: this is the medical examination carried out on the person concerned for the first time or when more than five years have elapsed since the date of the last medical examination for embarkation at sea; then there are periodic medical examinations: the cases not covered in the previous section.

The assessments of musculoskeletal pathologies are very broad, but for the purposes of this paper we will focus on lumbar pathologies. The main elements to be assessed in order to determine whether or not it is a disabling pathology for work, the degree of affection, whether it is acute or chronic, and how this will affect the seafarer's quality of life and work expectancy.

The first element to be assessed will be the health survey part, where elements such as the following should be assessed:

1. Current job.
2. Length of service in the current job.
3. Duration of working day: < 1 hour 1-2 hours 2-4 hours 4-6 hours 6-8 hours > 8 hours.
4. d.Task content in load handling: Lift/Position/Push/Pull/Pull/Pull.
5. Is the task of handling loads repetitive? yes/no.
6. The time spent on load handling tasks is: sporadic/continuous.
7. The weight of the load is: <1 Kg, 1-3 Kg, 3-25 Kg, > 25 Kg.

8. Have you ever suffered from tendinitis or tenosynovitis? yes/no. If yes, where?

9. Have you had any serious fractures or trauma? yes/no. If yes, where?

10. Have you suffered or do you suffer from any of the following diseases? diabetes gout collagenosis hypothyroidism osteoporosis osteomalacia rheumatism.

11. Do you practice sport? yes/no.

12. Do you have any of the following symptoms? Such as: pain, weakness, cramps, numbness in hands.

13. In the last 12 months, have you experienced problems in...?

- back of neck shoulder (right/left) elbow (right/left) wrist-hand.

- (right/left) upper spine lower spine hip.

- (right/left) knee (right/left) ankle-foot (right/left).

14. In the last 12 months have you been on sick leave due to problems in the following areas?

- neck shoulder (right/left) elbow (right/left).

- wrist-hand (right/left) upper spine lower spine.

- hip (right/left) knee (right/left) ankle-foot (right/left).

The second point of study should be the clinical history, which should include sections such as:

a. Anamnesis.

   a. Have you suffered or do you suffer?

      o contractures, cramps, muscle fibre ruptures.

      o tendinitis, tenosynovitis, tendon ruptures and/or.

      o ligament injuries, sprains, bursitis.

      o arthrosis, arthritis, herniated discs.

      o fractures, cracks.

      o neurological injuries.

      o vasomotor disorders.

      o abdominal and/or inguinal hernias.

   b. Have you suffered or do you suffer?

      o diabetes mellitus (DM).

      o ischaemic heart disease.

      o high blood pressure.

      o Dyslipidaemia.

      o other diseases.

c. Medical treatments he is currently undergoing.

d. Accidents at work and/or occupational diseases suffered.

e. Tobacco use: yes/no/smoker. If yes: number of cigarettes/years of use.

f. Consumption of alcoholic beverages: yes/no/ex-consumer.

g. If yes: units/day years of consumption.

h. Family history of:

   o diabetes mellitus.

   o coronary heart disease.

   o coagulation disorders.

   o neoplasms.

i. Do you carry out extra-occupational activities requiring manual handling of loads: yes/no. If yes, which ones? If yes, which ones, how long?

b. Non-specific clinical examination. The variables included are:

   a. Weight.

   b. Size.

   c. Body mass index.

   d. Blood pressure (systolic and diastolic).

   e. Heart rate.

   f. cardiac auscultation.

   g. Pulmonary auscultation.

   h. Abdominal palpation (rule out hernias).

c. Specific clinical examination. *Lumbar spine:*

   i. Inspection. With the subject naked, observe spontaneous mobility, look for skin lesions, postural attitude (lumbar tilt attitude: possible disc herniation), loss of physiological lordosis.

   ii. Palpation and tender points. With the patient standing and the explorer seated, placing the fingers above the iliac crests and the thumbs on the midline of the spine (L4-L5 space). Palpation of the spinous processes is performed (lack of sacral or lumbar processes is suggestive of spina bifida, a palpable or visible gap between one process and the next may indicate spondylolisthesis - more frequent between L5 over S1 or L4 over L5). The posterior interapophyseal joints, the posterior surface of the coccyx should also be palpated (the only way to palpate the coccyx completely is by rectal palpation), the paravertebral muscles (it is advisable for the patient to lean the head back in order to relax the fascia covering these muscles) and the sacroiliac joints (pelvic expansion test - in the supine position press down on the outer edges of the pelvis - and pelvic compression test - in the lateral position press down on the iliac blade) looking for the presence of pain indicative, in the first instance, of sacroiliitis.

   iii.   Mobility. The normal angles of lumbar mobilisation are:

- bending: 60º.
- extension: 35-40º.
- lateral tilt: 30º.
- rotation: 20º.
- toe-floor distance: 0 cm.
- rigid patient > 30-40 cm.
- Schöber test: 5 cm or more.

d. A series of exploratory physical tests or manoeuvres should be applied such as:
- Acromioclavicular Joint Manoeuvre
- Jobe manoeuvre.
- Patte's manoeuvre.
- Gerber manoeuvre.
- Yocum manoeuvre.
- Hawkins manoeuvre.
- Palm-up test or palm-up test.
- Proof of apprehension.

e. Management of musculoskeletal pathologies.
Management of the pathologies will be highly dependent on the acute or chronic conditions as appropriate to the individual seafarer. Injuries can be treated with NSAIDs, steroids, low level opioids and others. Depending on the injury, it will require rest, medical imaging tests and surgical procedures, depending on the case.

Bibliographical references.

1. Occupational Medicine. Protocols and action practices. Vicente MªT, Ramírez MªV, Murcia JJ. Letrera Publicaciones S.L. Bilbao, 2.008.

2. Mestré, Fernando. Protocol to be applied in medical examinations for embarkation related to the manual handling of loads. Expert Programme in Maritime Health. UCA, Spain.

3. Royal Decree 1696/2007, of 14 December, which regulates medical examinations for maritime embarkation.

4. Royal Decree 487/1.997 of 14 April 1997 on Minimum Health and Safety Provisions for the Manual Handling of Loads involving risks.

On-board assistance cases and others. Telemedicine.

Author: Hannah Diermissen Rodríguez
Email: hannahdiermissen@gmail.com

One of the main drawbacks in the maritime area is that in many cases medical assistance must be provided by tele-consultation, either by radio or, if there is a satellite signal, telepresence conditions may be available.

Telemedicine means medicine at a distance. In this sense, it encompasses several aspects of medical practice: diagnosis and treatment, but also health education, as long as they are carried out at a distance. Telematic technologies have evolved with the emergence and development of telecommunications, using technologies such as telegraphy, radiophony, telephone, satellite communications, cable, internet, the approaches given to this activity are aimed at developing three fundamental applications:

i. Healthcare telemedicine: this encompasses all activities related to the diagnosis and treatment of pathological processes. Within this branch of telemedicine, a series of variants can be distinguished with points in common: tele-assistance, tele-monitoring, teleconsultation between doctors.

ii. Administrative telemedicine: this type includes patient appointment programmes by telephone; telephone request/authorisation of complementary tests (analysis, radiology, etc.); archiving and shared access to medical records at the health centre, so that each doctor can access information on their patient at all times; exchange of electronic information between professionals; etc.

iii. Tele-training: allows the updating of the knowledge of health personnel (non-classroom courses) and the dissemination of informative content for citizens (information campaigns and health alerts).

There are many radio-medical centres in the world and the official health guides that all ships must carry and different nautical or maritime medicine manuals refer to their activity and the care they can provide. It could be said that the results obtained from the use of telemedicine for the provision of radio-medical services and the existence of well-trained personnel on the ship, together with the exploitation of tele-medical techniques and increasing cooperation between radio-medical centres around the world will achieve quality medical care everywhere.

Recommendation 106 of the International Labour Organisation (I.L.O.) is the first official document that sets out in detail what radio medical assistance to seafarers should look like. This document states that it should be free of charge, available and continuous, around the clock. The centre providing the telemedicine service must have a specialist available whenever necessary. An example of such a centre is the Sahlgrenska University Hospital in Gothenburg, Sweden, which is one of the largest hospitals in Europe and has been providing support and advice to ships all over the world since 1922.

Sahlgrenska is also the international reference hospital for the Swedish Maritime Administration, which in turn is the competent authority for setting the statutes, rules and regulations regarding medical care and medical kits on ships.

In the case of Spain, the Spanish Radio-Medical Centre can be contacted in the following ways: telephone: + 34.91.310.34.75, radio: if the coastal station is Spanish, ask for "medical consultation" and they will connect with the Centre directly (the C.R.M.E. is the medical centre of reference, as we have already indicated). If the radio station is foreign, just ask for a conference with the C.R.M.E. telephone number.

Depending on the problem for which the C.R.M.E. has been called, the physician may make three decisions:

1. Treatment of the sick person on board his ship: the case is not serious.

2. Disembarkation of the crew member at the next arrival: the severity of the case and the means on board allow the case to be monitored from the medical centre: infectious, endocrine, mental, nervous system, cardio-circulatory system, respiratory, digestive system, genitourinary, skin, musculoskeletal, symptoms/signs, accidents.

3. Evacuation of the patient: the seriousness of the case or the lack of adequate means of treatment make it advisable not to keep the patient on board any longer.

However, what are the benefits of using telemedicine instead of traditional medicine?

There are a number of advantages that are easily understood as cost savings and benefits for the population:

o Savings in travel costs for patients to health centres.

o Savings in travel costs for health personnel to visit widely scattered populations.

o Reduced hospitalisation costs by reducing hospital stays for those patients who can recover at home under remote medical supervision.

o To name but a few.

However, it is important to remember that telemedicine should not be the first option in the case of telemedicine if the physical resources are available to be able to carry out the medical act adequately. Teleconsultation is a valuable resource, but it is not a substitute for doctor-patient contact.

Bibliographical references.

1. Goethe W. Manual of Nautical Medicine. ISM. Spriger-Verlag Ibérica. Barcelona, 1992.

2. International Medical Guide on Board. World Health Organization. Geneva, 1989.

3. Health Guide on board. Instituto Social de la Marina. Madrid, 2001.

4. Sánchez-Caro J, Abellán F. Telemedicina y protección de datos sanitarios (aspectos legales y éticos). Ed. Comares. Granada.

5. Stanberry B. Legal and ethical issues in European telemedicine. European Telemedicine 1999.

6. Wootton R. Telemedicine: an introduction. European Telemedicine 1999 .

Traveller's medicine and rescue at sea.

Author: Hannah Diermissen Rodríguez
Email: hannahdiermissen@gmail.com

In the following, we will discuss two tropical diseases that are often difficult to manage for crew members, officers and passengers. We will review the general characteristics of dengue fever and yellow fever, which are the most prevalent tropical diseases in developing and third world countries.

Tropical diseases are infectious diseases prevalent in tropical and subtropical regions of the world. These territories are characterised by hot and humid climates and are, for the most part, socially, economically and sanitarily underdeveloped regions. The risk of acquiring infections will depend on several factors, such as the purpose of travel, the itinerary, the quality of accommodation, hygiene, sanitation and the traveller's own behaviour.

The main routes of transmission of tropical diseases are: food and water, vectors: yellow fever and dengue fever, animals which cause zoonoses, to name a few.

Dengue fever.

In its aetiological origin it is a disease caused by the dengue virus, a flavivirus, of which there are 4 related serotypes: Den-1, Den-2, Den-3 and Den-4. It is transmitted by the Aedes aegypti mosquito, which bites during daylight hours; it can present in 3 clinical forms:

i.   Dengue fever: an acute febrile illness manifested by the sudden onset of fever, followed by generalised symptoms and sometimes a macular skin rash. Patients recover within a few days.

ii. Dengue haemorrhagic fever: characterised by acute onset of fever followed by other symptoms such as thrombocytopenia, increased vascular permeability and haemorrhagic manifestations.

iii. Dengue shock syndrome: very rare, but causes severe hypotension requiring urgent treatment to correct hypovolaemia.

It is widespread in tropical and subtropical regions of Central and South America, Southeast and South Asia, as well as in Africa. For travellers, the risk is high in endemic areas and in areas affected by dengue epidemics. Treatment will range from mild symptom management to intensive care management for fluid and electrolyte replacement.

Yellow fever.

Yellow fever is caused by the yellow fever virus, an arbovirus belonging to the genus Flavivirus, which is transmitted by the bite of, among others, the Aedes aegypti mosquito during daylight hours. The vectors that cause this disease can be found in the forests of South America. The yellow fever virus infects both humans and monkeys, so it can also be a zoonosis. Infectious mosquitoes may bite humans entering forested areas, resulting in sporadic cases or small outbreaks. In urban areas, human-to-human infection is transmitted by mosquitoes, resulting in large epidemics of yellow fever in densely populated areas.

The disease is difficult to recognise in the early stages and diagnosis is made by blood test. Most infections cause an acute illness that develops in 2 phases: A first phase with fever, muscle pain, headache, chills, anorexia, nausea and/or vomiting, often with bradycardia, and a second phase with recurrence of fever, jaundice, abdominal pain, vomiting and haemorrhagic manifestations. By international standards, yellow fever is an internationally notifiable disease.

Yellow fever virus is endemic in some tropical areas of Africa and Central and South America, and travellers are at risk of exposure in all areas where yellow fever is endemic. The highest risk occurs in jungle and forested areas.

Vaccination is mandatory for entry into some countries. Regardless of this requirement, vaccination is recommended for all travellers to endemic areas, and is only administered in authorised vaccination centres, where the International Certificate of Vaccination is issued and is legally valid for 10 years from 10 days after the first dose, and immediately upon revaccination. However, when vaccination against yellow fever is contraindicated for medical reasons, it is necessary to carry a medical certificate of exemption issued by the international vaccination centres.

Treatment will depend on each case and precautions should be taken to avoid mosquito bites during the day and at night.

Bibliographical references.

1. African trypanosomiasis (sleeping sickness). Revised: 16 July 2022. Available at: www.who.int/mediacentre/factsheets/fs259/en

2. Bell R. Tropical Medicine. 4th ed. Leeds: Blackwell Science Ltd.; 1995.

3. Infectious diseases of potential risk to travellers. Revised: 14 July 2022. Available at: http://www.msc.es/profesionales/saludPublica/sanidadExterior/salud/viajesInter/cap5htm

4. Yellow fever. Revised: 16 July 2022. Available at: http://www.who.int/topics/yellow_fever/es/

CHAPTER IV. OCCUPATIONAL RISK PREVENTION, SAFETY, REGULATIONS AND EMERGENCIES APPLIED TO MARITIME MEDICINE

Occupational hazards and maritime emergencies.

Author: William Gutiérrez Sandí
Email: wgutierrezs@hotmail.com

Origins of maritime rescue .

The birth of the RNLI .

It is important to remember how maritime rescue systems were born. It was in 1823 when William Hillary (1774-1847) published in England a pioneering proclamation under the title: "*An appeal to the British nation on behalf of Mankind to form a National Institution for the Salvage of Life and Property in Shipwrecks*". Later, in 1852, William Hillary created the

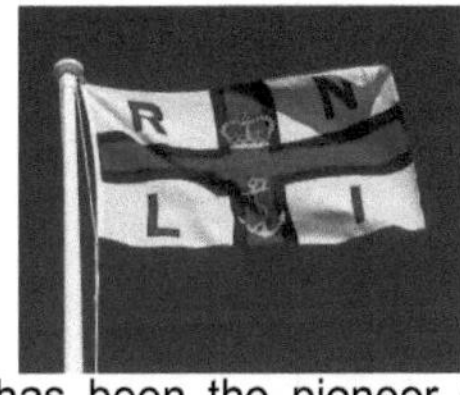

Royal National Lifeboat Institution (RNLI), which has been the pioneer of **Maritime Rescue in the World** and has had the constancy to remain operative today with the same spirit that inspired Sir William Hillary.

Following the English model in Europe and French and/or English colonies, the same trend was followed in the creation of charitable, non-governmental societies to help shipwrecked persons, most of these were diluted or became parastatal agencies. The Hamburg Convention was an event that led to investment in maritime rescue and anti-pollution infrastructures, as well as in means of controlling ship traffic along the coasts in different parts of Europe. In England, for example, although the RNLI has survived, HM Coastguard was created in 1822 as the Maritime Prosecution Service, which was later integrated into the Royal Navy in 1850, before merging with the Marine Pollution Control Unit in 1923 and establishing the Coastguard Agency as it is known today. In addition, the Coastguard Control Centres (MRCC) co-ordinate not only their environment, but also those of the RNLI, as well as those of the Royal Navy and Royal Air Force. There is also a volunteer corps called the Auxiliary Coastguard.

Let us now look at the case of Germany where, in 1860, the organisation of maritime salvage was set up with a patron provided by the RNLI and the "Deutchen Gesellschaft zur Rettung Schiffbrüchiger (DGzRS)" was born. Also, in France in 1865, the "Société Centrale de Sauvetage des Naufrages" was founded, which no longer exists today, although the "Société Nationale de Sauvetage en Mer" still exists.

Sociedad Española de Salvamento de Náufragos" (SESN) the Spanish RNLI .

Another important salvage society developed in Spain from 1859 onwards, and was preceded by local societies. Thus, on 19 December 1880, the unified "Sociedad Española de Salvamento de Náufragos" (SESN) was founded. The SESN gradually declined in its activity and in the progressive loss of means that would enable it to meet the needs of a maritime country like Spain, and the Spanish Civil War put an end to it.

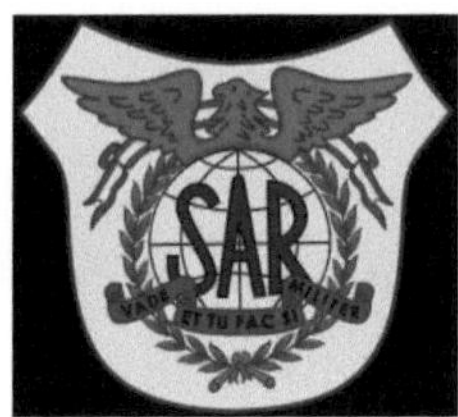

In the period from 1940 to 1970. As part of the Air Force, the "Air Rescue Service (SAR)" was created, which with the acronym SAR also stood for the international acronym "search and rescue". The SAR, created in 1955, still exists today and has complemented the work of the Navy in the beginning and now the Sociedad Estatal de Salvamento Marítimo. In 1970, the Undersecretariat of the Merchant Navy proposed the participation of the Spanish Red Cross in the provision of rescue services for shipwrecked persons, and in 1971 the "Provisional Rules of Operation of the Red Cross at Sea" (CRM) were published, while the Spanish Society for the Rescue of Shipwrecked Persons (SESN) was integrated into the CRM in 1972 to provide assistance for this type of project.

The Spanish state acquired international commitments such as the International Convention on the High Seas (1958), which required the establishment of a SAR service, the Convention for the Safety of Life at Sea (1974), which also required States to establish and notify a SAR service, and the International Convention on Maritime Rescue (1979), which the Spanish government was slow to sign as it imposed means of control and assistance that Spain did not have. In addition, the United Nations Convention on the Law of the Sea (1982) was signed, which explicitly obliged Spain to establish a SAR service.

However, it was the signing of the State Ports and Merchant Navy Act in 1992, which brought about the creation of SASEMAR (Sociedad de Salvamento y Seguridad Marítima) under the principle of coordination that made the difference in the model of care for seafarers in emergency situations. Article 90 of the Ports Act stated that the purpose of SASEMAR was to provide search, rescue and rescue services, prevention and fight against pollution of the marine environment, control and assistance to maritime traffic, towage and auxiliary vessel services and complementary services to the aforementioned.

Sociedad de Salvamento y Seguridad Marítima (SASEMAR) .

Structure of SASEMAR .

SASEMAR is a public business entity attached to the Ministry of Public Works through the DGMM. It was created in 1992 by the aforementioned Law on Ports and came into operation in Spain in 1993. It is the Spanish body for the global coordination of SAR services, as required by the Hamburg Convention of 1979. In addition, the emergency communication systems included in the GMDSS (radio, radio beacons, etc.) and the emergency telephone 900-202-202 allow seafarers, fishermen, pleasure boats, etc., to establish contact 24 hours a day.

The SASEMAR Operations Directorate is the basic body for managing maritime traffic, the provision of SAR services and the prevention and fight against marine pollution. The National Rescue Coordination Centre (CNCS), which in turn coordinates the more than 20 centres distributed along the Spanish coast, is directly related to this Directorate.

The categories of these are:

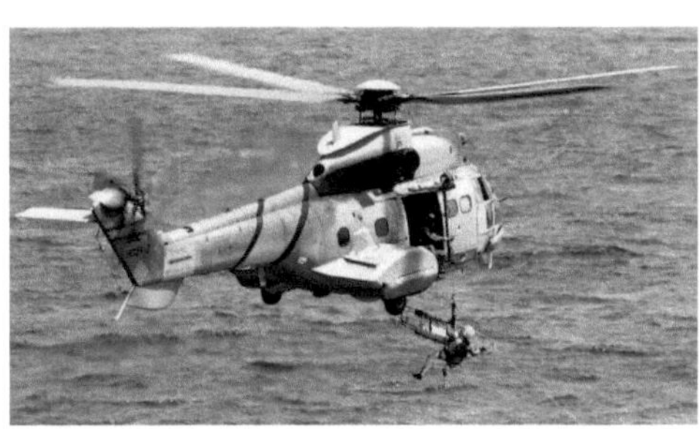

- ZONAL CENTRES (CZCS)

- REGIONAL CENTRES (CRCS)

- LOCAL CENTRES (CLCS)

SASEMAR has "Helimer" helicopters for its search and rescue operations, as well as fixed-wing aircraft, and two types of maritime units: rescue vessels or deep-sea tugs, some of which are exclusive, and the "Salvamar".

The control towers .

The Control Towers or MRCC started to be installed in Spain very late, in 1987 it was the one in Tarifa-Traffic that started to control the separation device working in a network of centres distributed throughout the Spanish territory.

National Rescue Plans (NSP) .

SASEMAR has been developing various "National Plans for Special Services for the Rescue of Human Life at Sea and the Fight against Pollution of the Marine Environment", generally known as National Rescue Plans (PSN) and structured in six programmes:

1. Rescue and pollution response resources programme.

2. Peripheral Centres Programme.

3. Training and prevention programme.

4. Research and innovation programme.

5. Coordination programme.

6. Fishing Vessel Safety Programme.

The NSP establishes that, in order to deal with possible accidents due to spills or spillages, Maritime Rescue needs to have sufficient action material (booms, oil suction devices, etc.) at strategic points or bases. The PSN inventory for 2009 was as follows:

i.   14 own vessels (10 tugboats and 4 multipurpose vessels).

ii.   1 collection vessel with a capacity of 3,000 m3 (chartered), which, together with the rest of the means, will increase the collection capacity of polluting products to 7,300 m3.

iii.   55 "Salvamares" vessels, 16 of them newly built.

iv.   10 multi-purpose fast vessels ~25-30 m, all of them newly built, a new model being added to the maritime fleet for the first time.

v.   10 helicopters, of which 8 will be newly built and owned, and 2 will be leased.

vi.   new-build fixed-wing aircraft.

vii.   strategic bases for rescue and marine pollution response and 5 local bases.

viii.   bases of underwater performance.

Traffic protection and control structures in Europe .

In relation to this issue, there are several structures that carry out pollution prevention and international representation, resource management: maritime traffic control, maritime traffic service, etc., marine pollution control in the European Union. Piniella (2009) in his work: The Safety of Maritime Transport mentions several of these structures and organisations that have a role at European level.

Table 02. Pollution prevention, traffic resource management and marine pollution control tables.

A) PREVENCIÓN DE LA CONTAMINACIÓN y REPRESENTACIÓN INTERNACIONAL

PAISES	ORGANO COMPETENTE			
	NOMBRE	TIPO DE INSTITUCIÓN	DEPENDENCIA DIRECTA	DEPENDENCIA MINISTERIAL
ALEMANIA	Subdirección de Contaminación Marina (Organismo Normativo) SBOE – Agencia Federal para el control de la Contaminación Marina (Actuación Preventiva)	Administración Central Sociedad Estatal	Dirección General del Transporte Marítimo	Ministerio de Transporte Ministerio de Medio Ambiente
FRANCIA	Direction des Affaires Maritimes et des Gents de Mer	Administración Central	Servicios Centrales del Ministerio Secretariado General del Mar	Ministerio de Equipamiento, Transportes y Vivienda Secretariado General del Mar
ITALIA	Ministerio de Medio Ambiente (Org. Normativo) Guardia Costiera (nivel ejecutivo)	Administración Central Organismo Autónomo		Ministerio de Transportes y Navegación Ministerio de Medio Ambiente
REINO UNIDO	Unidad de Control de la Polución marina (MPCU)	Agencia Estatal	Her Majesty Coast Guard (HMCG)	Departamento de Medio Ambiente, Transportes y Regiones
ESPAÑA	Dirección General de la Marina Mercante	Administración Central	Ministerio de Fomento	Ministerio de Fomento

B) GESTIÓN DE RECURSOS: CONTROL TRÁFICO MARÍTIMO, SERV. TRÁFICO MARÍTIMO, etc.

| PAISES | ORGANO COMPETENTE | | | DEPENDENCIA MINISTERIAL |
	NOMBRE	TIPO DE INSTITUCIÓN	DEPENDENCIA DIRECTA	
ALEMANIA	Agencia Federal de Seguridad Marítima Länders	Agencia Federal	Dirección General del Transporte Marítimo	Ministerio de Transporte
FRANCIA	Direction des Affaires Maritimes et des Gents de Mer Direcciones Regionales de Asuntos Marítimos Centros Regionales (CROSS)	Administración Central Administración Regional	Prefecto Marítimo Colectividad Territorial	Ministerio de Equipamiento, Transportes y Vivienda Defensa
ITALIA	Guardia Costiera	Organismo Autónomo		Ministerio de Transportes y Navegación
REINO UNIDO	Channel Navigation Information System (CNIS)	Agencia Estatal	Her Majesty Coast Guard (HMCG)	Departamento de Medio Ambiente, Transportes y Regiones
ESPAÑA	Dirección General de la Marina Mercante Sociedad de Salvamento y Seguridad Marítima	Administración Central	Ministerio de Fomento	Ministerio de Fomento

C) LUCHA CONTRA LA CONTAMINACIÓN MARINA

| PAISES | ORGANO COMPETENTE | | | DEPENDENCIA MINISTERIAL |
	NOMBRE	TIPO DE INSTITUCIÓN	DEPENDENCIA DIRECTA	
ALEMANIA	SBOE – Agencia Federal para el control de la Contaminación Marina (Actuación Preventiva) ELG – National Spill Response Team – (Coordinación entre Gobierno Federal y Gobiernos Regionales – Länders-)	Administración Central	Dirección General del Transporte Marítimo	Ministerio de Transporte Ministerio de Medio Ambiente
FRANCIA	Prefectura Marítima Divisions Actino de l'etat en Mer	Administración Central	Secretariado General del Mar	Ministerio de Equipamiento, Transportes y Vivienda Ministerios de Medio Ambiente, Defensa e Interior
ITALIA	Guardia Costiera (nivel ejecutivo)	Organismo Autónomo		Ministerio de Transportes y Navegación Ministerio de Medio Ambiente
REINO UNIDO	Unidad de Control de la Polución marina (MPCU)	Agencia Estatal	Her Majesty Coast Guard (HMCG)	Departamento de Medio Ambiente, Transportes y Regiones
ESPAÑA	Dirección General de la Marina Mercante Sociedad de Salvamento y Seguridad Marítima	Administración Central	Subsecretaria de Fomento	Ministerio de Fomento

Source: Piniella (2009) The Security of Maritime Transport

Bibliographical references.

1. IMO (2002). SOLAS: International Convention for the Safety of Life at Sea, 1974, and its 1988 Protocol: 2000 Amendments in force in January and July 2002. Revised: 1 July 2022. Available at: https://labordoc.ilo.org/discovery/fulldisplay/alma993679053402676/41ILO_INST:41ILO_V2

2. IMO (2022). Frequently Asked Questions on the Maritime Labour Convention. Revised: 1 July 2022. Available at: https://www.ilo.org/global/standards/maritime-labour-convention-old/faq/WCMS_CON_TXT_ILS_MAR_FAQ_ES/lang--es/index.htm

3. Piniella, F (2009). Maritime Transport Safety, UCA, Cadiz, Spain.

International Convention for the Safety of Life at Sea (SOLAS 74/78). SEVIMAR (SOLAS).

Author: William Gutiérrez Sandí
Email: wgutierrezs@hotmail.com

What is SOLAS?

Although SOLAS 74 was signed in that year, 1974, it did not enter into force until six years later, on 25 May 1980, when the double condition of 50% GRT acceptance by the world fleet and a minimum of 25 contracting states was reached.

SOLAS is a convention for the safety of shipping which consists of thirteen articles setting out the legal principles that contracting governments agree to establish in order to enhance the safety of life at sea.

It consists of articles on the following topics:

1. On general obligations under the Convention.

2. The scope of application.

3. On national legislation and the need to list national bodies with authority over the subject matter of the Convention.

4. Cases of force majeure and emergencies in which ships are not subject to the Convention.

5. The relationship with the previous Conventions (terms of validity).

6. The amendment procedure (which we discussed earlier), signature for ratification, approval, accession and grace period.

7. The denunciation of the Convention.

8. The formal aspects of deposit, registration and language and official drafting translations.

The Convention is not limited to these thirteen articles, but also includes an Annex, structured in chapters, parts, sections and rules. This annex is the real technical body of the Convention and the tool to be used by professionals in shipbuilding, navigation and commercial operation.

The SOLAS convention was born out of the need to protect the safety of seafarers, because sea voyages always involve danger. The rules concerning the safety of ships differ in scope from country to country. It was around 1855 that efforts to draw up international rules on ship safety began with the introduction of the International Code of Signals by the British Board of Trade, and in 1863, when the "Rule of the Road at Sea" was created, following an international agreement aimed at preventing collisions between ships.

The Titanic disaster in 1912 was the trigger for the development of international rules governing the safety of life at sea.

On that occasion, 1,503 people lost their lives. As a result, the United Kingdom convened a conference of nations with a maritime tradition with the aim of creating an international convention for the safety of life at sea, which was created in 1914 and is known as the SOLAS (Safety Of Life At Sea) Convention of 1914 (SEVIMAR).

The main objective of the SOLAS Convention was the creation of minimum standards for the construction, equipment and use of ships, compatible with their safety. At the same time, it establishes that flag states are also responsible for ensuring that ships flying their flag comply with the provisions of the convention, and thus for issuing a series of certificates which guarantee the safety of the ship and its crew.

The provisions concerning oversight empower contracting governments to inspect the ships of other contracting states if there are reasonable grounds to believe that a given ship and its equipment do not comply with the requirements of the convention, referred to as "port state control".

In the updated version of the SOLAS Convention, it contains provisions laying down general obligations, as well as amendment procedures and other provisions. It is structured in 14 chapters in an annex.

The following is an overview of the scope of the chapters of the agreement:

Chapters of the SOLAS Convention.

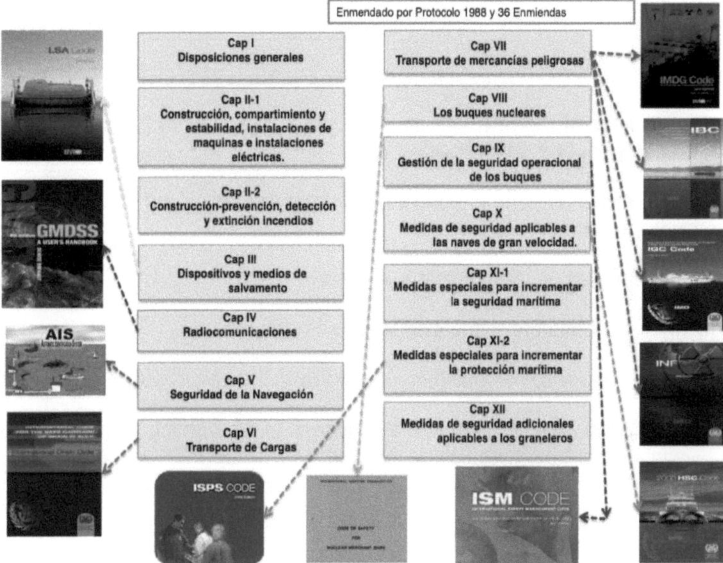

Figure 04. Diagram showing the chapters of the 1998 SOLAS protocol and the applicable amendments.
Source: https://marygerencia.com/2011/01/21/convenio-internacional/

Chapter I. General Provisions.

The chapter discusses the general rules for the survey of the various types of ships, the issuance of documents certifying the ship as compliant with the requirements of the Convention, as well as aspects of the supervision of ships in ports of other Contracting Governments.

Chapter II-1. Construction - Compartmentalisation and stability, machinery installations and electrical installations.

The subdivision of passenger ships into watertight compartments is to be so designed that following a hull damage event the ship remains afloat and in a stable position. Include requirements for watertight integrity and bilge circuit arrangements for passenger ships as well as stability requirements for passenger and cargo ships.

Chapter II-2. Fire prevention, detection and extinguishing.

Covering fire safety issues applicable to all ships, these cover measures in relation to passenger ships, cargo ships and tankers.

These provisions set out principles such as:

- The division of the ship into main and vertical zones by means of isolated structural boundary bulkheads.

- Separation of accommodation spaces from the rest of the ship by insulated structural boundary bulkheads.

- Restricted use of combustible materials.

- Detection of any fire in the area where it originates.

- Containment and extinguishing of any fire in the space where it originates.

- Protection of means of escape and access to fire-fighting positions; prompt availability of fire extinguishing devices.

- Minimisation of the risk of ignition of cargo gases.

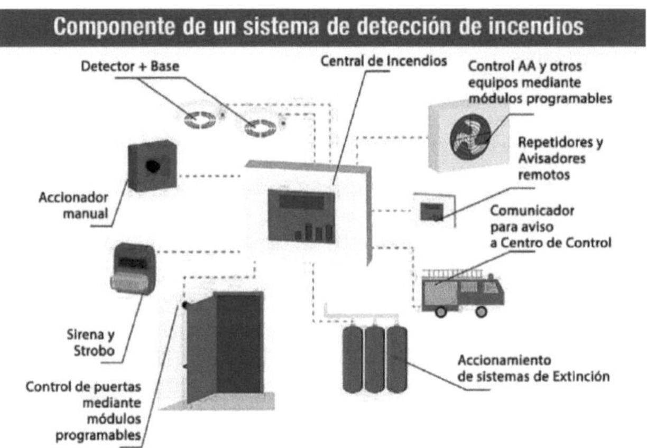

Figure 05. Example of an image depicting the components of a fire detection system. **Source:** https://revistainnovacion.com/nota/10467/nociones_basicas_de_un_sistema_de_deteccion_de_incendios/

Chapter III. Rescue devices and means of rescue.

The chapter lays down provisions concerning life-saving appliances and arrangements, including requirements for lifeboats, rescue boats and lifejackets depending on the type of ship.

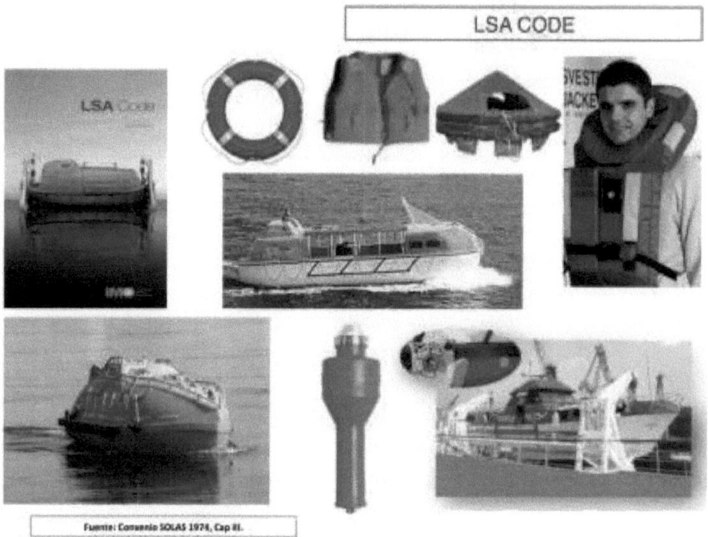

Figure 06. Examples of safety devices covered by the SOLAS Convention. SOLAS Convention 1974, Chapter III.
Source: https://marygerencia.com/2011/01/21/convenio-internacional/

The International Life-Saving Appliance Code (IDS Code) lays down specific technical requirements for life-saving appliances, which under Regulation 34 are mandatory in that all life-saving appliances and means of rescue shall comply with the applicable requirements of the IDS Code.

Chapter IV. Radiocommunications.

The chapter details the Global Maritime Distress and Safety System (GMDSS). All passenger and cargo ships of 300 gross tonnage and above engaged on international voyages are required to carry equipment designed to improve the chances of rescue following an accident. This regulation establishes the need for satellite-based radio locator beacons (EPIRBs), search and rescue responders (SARs) used for the location of ships or survival craft. This chapter is closely linked to the Radio Regulations of the International Telecommunication Union.

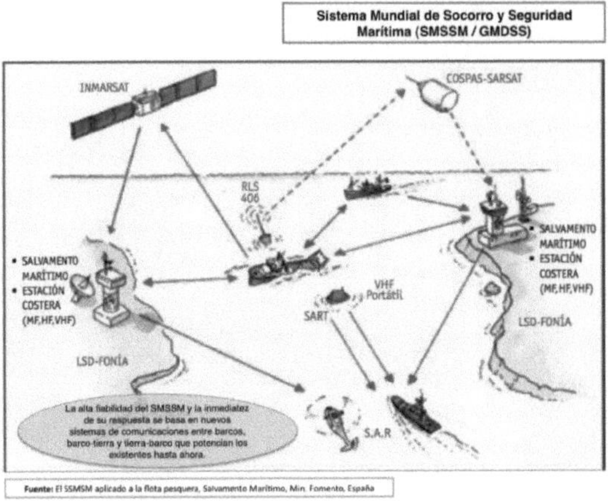

Figure 07. Graphical scheme of the Global Maritime Distress and Safety System (GMDSS). GMDSS applied to the fishing flora, Salvamento marítimo, Min. Fomento, Spain.
Source: https://marygerencia.com/2011/01/21/convenio-internacional/

Chapter V. Safety at sea.

Chapter V establishes safety of navigation services which Contracting Governments are required to provide. This chapter sets out provisions of an operational nature generally applicable to all ships engaged on all types of voyages.

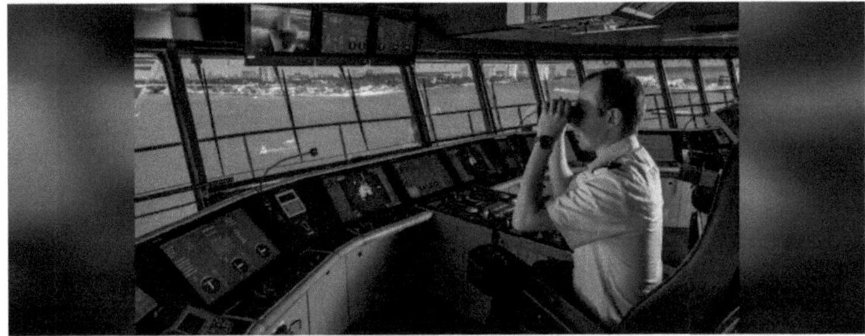

Figure 08. Example of a command post for safety management in navigation.
Source: https://trends.nauticexpo.es/project-331247.html

It covers such matters as the maintenance of meteorological services for ships; the ice-watch service; the organisation of traffic; and the provision of search and rescue services. It also stipulates the obligation of masters to render assistance to those in distress, and the obligation of contracting governments to take measures to ensure that all ships are adequately and competently manned from a safety point of view.

The carriage of voyage data recorders (VDR) and automatic identification systems (AIS) on board ships is regulated on a mandatory basis.

Chapter VI - Carriage of cargoes.

This chapter regulates the types of cargoes (except bulk liquids and gases) "which, because of the particular hazards they pose to ships and persons on board, may require special precautions".

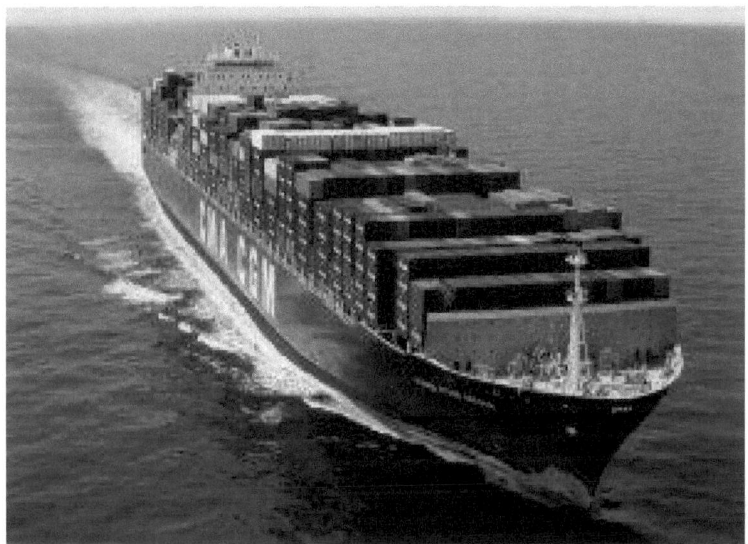

Figure 09. Example of a merchant vessel engaged in the carriage of cargo goods.
Source: https://grupoberistain.com/principales-buques-de-carga-en-el-transporte-maritimo/

Its rules lay down requirements for the stowage and securing of cargo and cargo units, such as containers.

Chapter VII - Transport of dangerous goods.

In this chapter, the rules are in three parts:

Part A: - Transport of dangerous goods in packages, containing provisions on classification, packaging, marking, labelling and placarding, documents and stowage of dangerous substances.

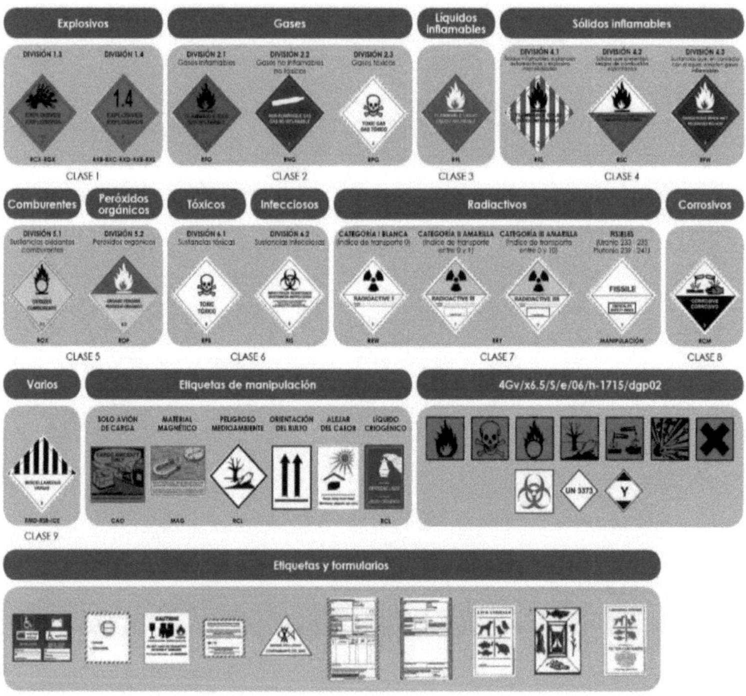

Figure 10. Hazard labels, handling, markings and dangerous goods forms.
Source: https://rellenardocumento.com/permiso-adr/

> *Part A-1:* Carriage of solid dangerous goods in bulk, for which document, stowage and segregation requirements are laid down for these goods, and for which reporting requirements are laid down for occurrences involving dangerous goods.
>
> *Part B:* sets out requirements for the construction and equipment of ships carrying dangerous liquid chemicals in bulk and requires chemical tankers to comply with the International Chemical Tanker Code (IBC Code).
>
> *Part C:* lays down requirements for the construction and equipment of ships carrying liquefied gases in bulk and provides that gas carriers shall comply with the International Gas Carrier Code (IGC Code).

Part D: establishes special requirements for the carriage of irradiated nuclear fuel, plutonium and high-level waste in packages on board ships, and also provides that ships carrying such items shall comply with the International Code for the Safe Carriage of Irradiated Nuclear Fuel, Plutonium and High-Level Waste in Packages on Board Ships (INF Code).

The chapter provides that the transport of dangerous goods shall be carried out in accordance with the relevant requirements of the International Maritime Dangerous Goods Code (IMDG Code).

Chapter VIII. Nuclear vessels.

Chapter VIII lays down the basic requirements for nuclear-powered ships and deals in particular with radiological hazards.

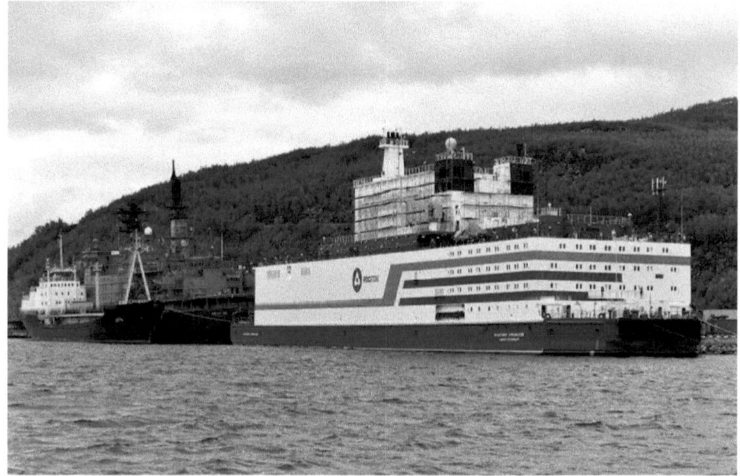

Figure 11. Example of a ship using nuclear power as a power source.
Source: https://hardwaresfera.com/noticias/internet/nuclear-tras-un-ano-la-central-nuclear-flotante-akademik-lomonosov-ha-llegado-a-la-ciudad-rusa-de-pevek/

In addition, its requirements refer to the detailed and comprehensive Code of Safety for Nuclear Merchant Ships, which was adopted by the IMO Assembly in 1981.

Chapter IX. Management of the operational safety of ships.

Chapter IX establishes a mandatory International Safety Management (ISM) Code, which requires the shipowner or any other person who has assumed responsibility for the ship. A safety management system must be established.

Chapter X. Safety measures applied to high speed craft.

This chapter makes the International Safety Code for High Speed Craft (HSC Code) mandatory.

Chapter XI. Special measures to enhance maritime safety and security.

Chapter XI-1. Special measures to enhance maritime safety.

It clarifies requirements relating to the authorisation of recognised organisations (responsible for carrying out surveys and inspections on behalf of Administrations); enhanced surveys; the system of assigning an IMO number to ships for their identification; and port State control of operational requirements.

Chapter XI-2. Special measures to enhance maritime security.

Regulation XI-2/3 of this chapter provides for the implementation of the International Ship and Port Facility Security Code (ISPS Code). Part A of the ISPS Code is mandatory and Part B provides guidance on how best to comply with the mandatory requirements.

Chapter XII. Safety measures applicable to bulk carriers.

Structural requirements for bulk carriers of 150 m in length and over are laid down as safety regulations in this chapter.

Chapter XIII - Verification of compliance.

It establishes the binding nature of the fulfilment of the responsibilities acquired under this convention by all member states.

The chapter provides for the introduction of verification audit systems that will serve to account for such compliance to the IMO.

Chapter XIV. Safety measures for ships operating in polar waters.

Ships operating for polar waters have a range of design, construction, equipment, operational, training, search and rescue and environmental protection requirements for ships operating in these waters which surround the two poles.

They also provide ships with the means to preserve human life at sea in these extreme temperatures and weather conditions.

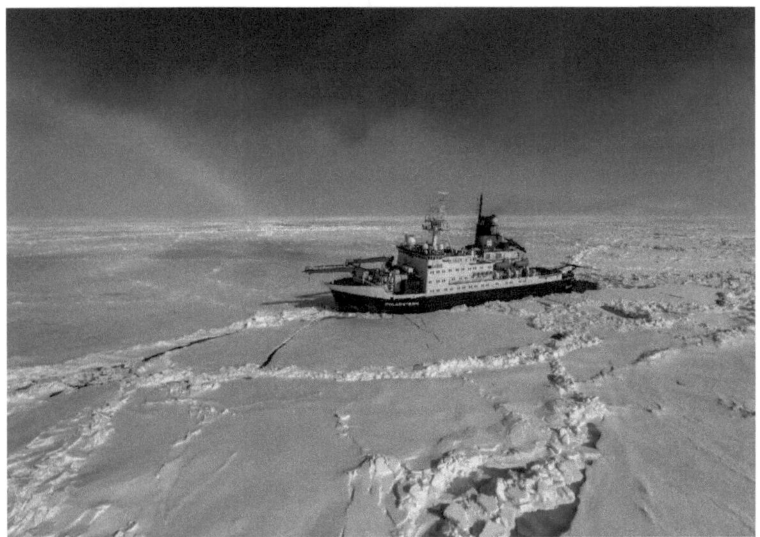

Figure 12. Example of a vessel used for transport on routes in polar regions.
Source: https://www.agenciasinc.es/Noticias/El-yodo-es-el-segundo-principal-responsable-de-la-destruccion-de-ozono-en-el-Artico

Concerning amendments.

The 1974 convention has been amended several times with a view to keeping it up to date. The amendments adopted by the Maritime Safety Committee (MSC) are contained in resolutions, covering issues related to shippers, carriers, and terminal ports. For operational purposes, the UN agency that regulates shipping, the International Maritime Organisation, has recommended that a practical approach be adopted during the first months of implementation of the new regulations.

Bibliographical references.

1. IMO (2002). SOLAS: International Convention for the Safety of Life at Sea, 1974, and its 1988 Protocol: 2000 Amendments in force in January and July 2002. Revised: 1 July 2022. Available at: https://labordoc.ilo.org/discovery/fulldisplay/alma993679053402676/41ILO_INST:41ILO_V2

2. IMO (2022). Frequently Asked Questions on the Maritime Labour Convention. Revised: 1 July 2022. Available at: https://www.ilo.org/global/standards/maritime-labour-convention-old/faq/WCMS_CON_TXT_ILS_MAR_FAQ_ES/lang--es/index.htm

CHAPTER V. PRINCIPLES OF PHYSIOLOGY, CRITERIA, REQUIREMENTS FOR ASSESSING FITNESS TO DIVE AND SOME EMERGENCY PATHOLOGIES IN THE MARITIME FIELD

Diving physiology and gas physics as applied to diving.

Author: William Gutiérrez Sandí
Email: wgutierrezs@hotmail.com

Diving physiology.

As the study material indicates, the aquatic environment presents very different environmental conditions from those on land, which is why the human body must make physiological variations to adapt to the aquatic environment during immersions, given that in water there are aggressive conditions that can be life-threatening.

Changes in vision.

Vision is one of the systems that is affected in the first way, as light enters the water it loses intensity due to three factors: reflection, absorption and dispersion, now the phenomenon of refraction occurs when changing from one medium to another of different density, that is to say, the light changes direction when it enters the water. The transmitted light is scattered to a greater or lesser degree depending on the type of water and its turbidity.

The extinction of light in water is due to absorption and scattering. As the light penetrates the water, it decreases due to absorption. Sunlight is made up of radiation of different wavelengths that make up the visible spectrum. The absorption pattern is a function of the wavelength of the solar spectrum.

Thus, the red and orange radiations of the spectrum are more rapidly absorbed than the green, blue and violet ones. In the first few centimetres, the extremes of the visible, infrared and ultraviolet range are lost; between 5 and 10 metres, red disappears; at 30 metres, yellow disappears; at 40 metres, only green and blue are visible; and below this, the spectrum becomes progressively darker.

Therefore, it is possible to say that with depth, a series of problems associated with the ability to see, as well as the effect of hypermetropia, will appear. This is why, in summary, there will be a progressive decrease in light, a progressive disappearance of colours, a lack of contrast, a need for a water mask, since objects or bodies appear 1/3 larger, closer, as well as a reduction of ¼ of the visual field with depth.

Changes in hearing.

Sound conduction in water is more efficient than in air (1,500m/s compared to 330m/s). It is transmitted four times faster and can reach great distances. Consequently, it reaches both ears simultaneously, negating the main means of determining the direction of sound. Now underwater, hearing is done by bone conduction and sound localisation depends on differences in amplitude detected by bone conduction, so transmission is faster.

Changes in temperature.

It is important to remember that changes in the body's deep tissue temperature, or core temperature, remain constant except for febrile states to within ± 0.6 °C. However, body temperature is regulated by the balance between heat production and heat loss.

Recall that almost all of the heat produced in the body is generated in the deep organs, in particular the liver, heart, and brain, but also in the muscles during exercise. The heat generated passes from these organs and deep tissues to the skin, where it is lost to the environment. The skin, subcutaneous tissue and, in particular, adipose tissue act in a coordinated manner as the body's thermal insulator.

However, in the aquatic environment, which is colder than air and has a thermal conductivity 24 times higher than air and a specific heat 1,000 times higher than air, the conduction of body heat through the water is greatly increased, these characteristics cause a much faster cooling in the water than in the air. For this reason and to protect against hypothermia, the diver wears a wetsuit.

Changes in the cardiovascular system.

Diving activity produces a modification of physiological parameters in the cardiovascular system as we have studied. When the body comes into contact with water, e.g. the face, the frontal and periorbital skin receptors induce a vagal reflex, called the immersion reflex, which can occur even when swimming alone. This reflex, also known as the "diving reflex" by translation of the "diving reflex", is present in all aquatic mammals, and involves a reduction in oxygen consumption that allows them to perform prolonged immersions in apnoea, a condition that we humans, who are naturally adapted to the terrestrial environment, cannot physiologically perform in a natural way.

On the other hand, the effect of hydrostatic pressure and the decrease in body temperature causes a redistribution of blood flow from the caudal and abdominal part of the body to the intrathoracic circulation with a consequent increase in venous return and intrathoracic core volume. This increase in preload and afterload causes an increase in cardiac work which stimulates volumetric receptors in the right atrial wall and inhibits antidiuretic hormone production. This hormonal feedback loop coupled with elevated renal blood flow leads to increased water permeability in distal renal tubule cells and increased urinary water loss resulting in so-called immersion diuresis. In this situation, and in response to the body's response to central hypervolaemia, there is an increase in blood pressure that stimulates the carotid baroreceptors and inhibits the renin-angiotensin-aldosterone axis which, in addition to lowering blood pressure, reduces sodium absorption in the renal tubule. The process described above contributes to the aforementioned immersion diuresis that occurs in diving.

Changes in the respiratory system.

The changes in lung ventilation during scuba diving are determined by several factors: supply of a breathing mixture by the regulator at a slightly higher pressure than the medium which makes inspiration almost passive, an increase in dead space, an increase in breathing gas density, as well as an increase in external resistances to air exhalation. The use of the regulator increases the expiratory pressure required to overcome the resistance of the equipment. These changes lead to a decrease in vital capacity and total lung volume by 3-9% and a tendency to hypercapnia.

Laws of physics as applied to diving.

From the readings, the three pillars of diving physics are pressure, Archimedes' principle and the gas laws. The first explains the variation of pressure with depth, the second the phenomenon of buoyancy and the last the behaviour of gases with varying pressure.

Pressure is defined as the force acting perpendicularly on a unit area and is expressed by the following formula: $P = f/s$.

Atmospheric pressure is defined as the force exerted by the weight of atmospheric air on the earth's surface. Atmospheric pressure decreases with altitude as the amount of air above it decreases, and hence its weight.

Hydrostatic pressure is the pressure exerted by the weight of a fluid at rest on the walls of the vessel containing it or on the surface of the object immersed in it. It is cumulative; as the diver descends he has more water above him and therefore more of this water weight (pressure) affecting his entire body surface.

Stevin's law states that the pressure exerted by a liquid depends on the specific gravity of the liquid and the height from the free surface of the liquid.

the pressure at which a submerged object is located or absolute pressure is the sum of the atmospheric pressure at sea level and the hydrostatic pressure determined by the depth at which the object is located or relative pressure; Absolute pressure = atmospheric pressure + relative pressure P = Pa + Pr.

Units of measurement.

In the International System of Units (SI), the unit of pressure is the Pascal (Pa) and is equivalent to *Newton*, one Pascal = Newton /m2.

The first unit used to measure atmospheric pressure was the "millimetre of mercury" (mmHg) due to Torricelli's experiment, according to which by filling a 1 m long tube (closed at one end) with mercury and inverting it over a bucket filled with mercury, the column of mercury drops several centimetres, remaining static at a height of about 76 cm (760 mm) because the atmospheric pressure exerted on the surface of the mercury (and transmitted throughout the liquid) is the same as the atmospheric pressure, the mercury column drops several centimetres, remaining static at a height of about 76 cm (760 mm) because the atmospheric pressure exerted on the surface of the mercury (and transmitted throughout the liquid and in all directions) supports the mercury column. A standard pressure has since been adopted and is called the atmosphere (ata), which is the pressure that supports a 76 cm column of mercury.

The equivalence 1 between the atmosphere and the SI unit of pressure is: 1 ata = 101.325 Pa.

Therefore, for academic purposes it is important to remember that different fields of science use different units of pressure. In medicine we use mm Hg, in meteorology we use Bar, in mechanics we use Kg/cm2: $1\ ATTA \cong 1\ Bar \cong 1\ kg/cm2 \cong 10\ m\ columna\ de\ agua$.

The atmosphere (ata) is the unit of measurement of pressure used in diving.

Archimides' principle, buoyancy.

One consequence of hydrostatic pressure is that when we put a body in a liquid, the liquid exerts a pressure on all the forces in the body. However, as the pressure increases with depth, the pressure on the lower part of the body is greater than the pressure on the upper part.

This force known as buoyancy was studied by Archimedes who enunciated the principle that bears his name, Archimedes' Principle: "Any body totally or partially immersed in a fluid experiences an upward force called buoyancy equal to the weight of the fluid displaced by the body".

Main gas laws applied to diving.

The behaviour of all gases conforms to three laws, which relate the volume of a gas to its temperature and pressure:

Boyle-Mariotte law.

"At constant temperature, the volume of a gas varies inversely proportional to the absolute pressure". That is, at constant temperature, the volume of a gas decreases with increasing pressure and increases with decreasing pressure.

When descending in water, a body faces an additional increase in hydrostatic pressure of 1 ata every 10m. Solid or liquid bodies remain stable, but the volume of gases according to Boyle's Law is progressively reduced by the effect of pressure following an exponential curve.

Charles' law.

"At constant pressure, the volume of a gas is directly proportional to the change in absolute temperature".

Gay-Lussac's Law or Charles' 2nd Law.

"At constant volume the pressure of the gas is directly proportional to the temperature".

Dalton's Law.

"The total pressure exerted by a mixture of gases is the sum of the partial pressures of each of the components of the mixture".

Henry's Law.

Henry's law, essential in diving-related pathophysiology, which states: "At constant temperature, the amount of gas dissolved in a liquid is a direct function of the pressure it exerts on the liquid". Or in other words: "At constant temperature and in a saturated state, the amount of gas dissolved in a liquid is proportional to the partial pressure of the gas".

Decompression theory.

Henry's Law the amount of gas that a liquid is capable of incorporating into its solution depends on three factors: the pressure that the gas exerts on the liquid-gas interface; the time that the gas is breathed in; and the solubility of the gas in the liquid, which is constant if the temperature does not vary. Nowadays, depending on the type of diving, the equipment used and the depth, stops must be made to prevent the nitrogen present in the tissues from coming out abruptly and causing decompression sickness. In 1908 the physiologist John S. Haldane was contracted by the British Royal Navy to study and solve the problem of the "diver's disease", he generated the first tables that have served as a base for the ones that nowadays are like the international guideline, although there is a great variety of diving tables available. In Spain, diving tables derived from those of the US Navy are used for military, scientific and commercial divers and recreational diving.

Bibliographical references.

1. Desola, J. Scuba diving in childhood. Physiological considerations and suitability criteria. Apunts. Medicina de l'Esport. January 2006; 41(149), 34-38. Spain, Barcelona. 2006. Cited: 13 October 2022. Retrieved from: https://www.apunts.org/es-buceo-con-escafandra-autonoma-infancia--articulo-X0213371706889759

2. Ministry of Transport, Mobility and Urban Agenda. BOE. 6745. Real Decreto 550/2020, de 2 de junio, por el que se determinan las condiciones de seguridad de las actividades de buceo. Spain, Ministry of Transport, Mobility and Urban Agenda. Year of publication: 26 June 2020. Cited: 12 October 2022. Retrieved from: https://www.boe.es/eli/es/rd/2020/06/02/550

3. University of Cadiz. Criteria for the assessment of diver competence. Spain: UCA: Cited: 12 October 2022. Retrieved from: https://av03-ext.uca.es/moodle/pluginfile.php/43418/mod_resource/content/1/10.2.%20Criterios%20de%20valoraci%C3%B3n%20de%20la%20aptitud%20para%20buceadores.pdf

Criteria and requirements in the assessment of fitness for professional divers.

Author: William Gutiérrez Sandí
Email: wgutierrezs@hotmail.com

General.

Diving, whether professional or sport diving, takes place in a hostile environment, the underwater environment, where the use of technology is part of the requirements for its development, and therefore the health conditions of the people who practice it are of utmost importance.

At the Spanish level, the literature indicates two main guiding principles: first, the International Association of Diving Contractors (ADCI), whose objective is to promote the highest possible level of safety in the practice of commercial diving and underwater operations. To this end, it published in 2016 a Consensus of International Standards for Commercial Diving and Underwater Operations, and among its parts there is a section which refers to the medical and training requirements for diving personnel.

The second important actor is the Social Marine Institute (ISM), which is the governmental organisation managing the social security system that defined a Professional Diving Protocol in 2015, with the aim of being applied to all professional divers affiliated to the Special Regime for the Sea, in accordance with the requirements published in Royal Decree 550/2020, of 2 June 2022, which determines the safety conditions for diving activities for professionals who must be validated and accredited by the Spanish authorities. Previously, the regulation on this matter was scattered in different rules, among which Decree 2055/1969, of 25 September, regulating the exercise of underwater activities, and the Order of 14 October 1997 approving the safety rules for the exercise of underwater activities.

Therefore, Decree 550/2020 of 2 June 2022 was intended to update and unify these currently dispersed regulations, replacing them with an adequate regulation of the safety standards to be observed in the practice of diving activities. However, the coverage of this regulation dealt only with maritime safety issues. The spirit of the law, in this case of the royal decree, sought to regulate technical issues as little as possible, in order to allow, in the face of technological evolution, independence between the technical elements required and regulated, as well as the legal regulations, allowing divers, depending on their activity and specific environment, to comply with the European and international safety standards they consider most appropriate.

In addition, the Directorate General of the Merchant Navy reserved for itself the exercise of the functions required to safeguard maritime safety and human life at sea, for the protection of the people and other actors involved.

Important definitions for diving.

Royal Decree 550/2020, of 2 June 2022, defines a series of concepts which are copied verbatim from it in order to provide an overview of the basic elements involved in this activity. For the purposes of this Royal Decree, it is understood by:

1. Diving: an underwater activity in which a person is kept underwater in a hyperbaric environment either with the aid of apparatus or means allowing the exchange of a breathable gaseous mixture with the exterior, or any system that facilitates breathing, or without the aid of such apparatus, means or systems.

2. Diver: a person who is subjected to a hyperbaric environment for the purpose of diving.

3. Hyperbaric environment: an environment in which the ambient pressure is higher than atmospheric pressure.

4. Confined space means any space or environment in which there is only one point of entry and exit through which two divers cannot pass at the same time. Such a confined space may include, but is not limited to, a cave or wreck.

5. Emergency locator device: a device that allows the diver to be quickly located during the dive operation.

6. Partial pressure: is the pressure exerted by one gas on the total of the mixture. In a mixture of gases, the total pressure will be equal to the sum of the partial pressures of the gases that make up the mixture.

7. Air: binary breathing mixture of nitrogen and oxygen, where 78 per cent nitrogen, 21 per cent oxygen and 1 per cent trace gases are present. For decompression purposes, air shall be considered to contain 79 per cent nitrogen and 21 per cent oxygen.

8. Nitrox: gas containing a specific mixture of oxygen and nitrogen, capable of sustaining human life under appropriate diving or hyperbaric conditions. Nitrox is commonly referred to as a binary breathing mixture of nitrogen and oxygen when oxygen is present in a proportion greater than 21 per cent.

9. Trimix: gas containing a specific mixture of oxygen, helium and nitrogen, capable of sustaining human life under appropriate diving or hyperbaric conditions.

10. Heliox: gas containing a specific mixture of oxygen and helium, capable of sustaining human life under appropriate diving or hyperbaric conditions.

11. Umbilical: a system of flexible elements with adequate buoyancy, allowing the supply of breathing mixture and necessary services to the diver, depending on the type of equipment used.

12. Hyperbaric chamber: A pressurised enclosure intended for human occupancy, equipped with means to regulate the pressure differential between the inside and outside of the chamber. This enclosure shall be used both for the treatment of pathologies related to hyperbaric exposure and to perform or complete periods of surface decompression, both as part of diving operations.

13. Manual tool: those defined as such in the Technical Notes on Prevention of the National Institute for Safety and Health at Work (Instituto Nacional de Seguridad y Salud en el Trabajo).

14. Dive plan: document that includes all the planning and resources, both human and material, used in a diving operation. It should include the procedures to be followed in the event of a diving accident, as well as the evacuation of casualties to a medical centre of reference and to a hyperbaric chamber for treatment.

15. Diving system: any apparatus, device, device, equipment or installation that is used in a diving operation.

16. Non-saturation diving: a dive in a hyperbaric environment, where the exposure does not result in total saturation of the diver's tissues.

17. Saturation dive: a dive into a hyperbaric environment, the exposure of which results in total saturation of the diver's tissues.

18. Surface marker buoy: a buoy of a highly visible colour, which may contribute to its detection, flying the flag of the International Code of Signals "Alpha".

19. Scientific team: a group of people who dive in a hyperbaric environment to carry out a specific, duly authorised scientific study or project.

20. Auxiliary personnel to the scientific team: any diver who is not part of the scientific team, but who is necessary for the development of the activity.

21. Decompression table: structured set of decompression schedules or limits, usually arranged in increasing order of bottom time and depth.

22. Safety Diver: Diver participating in dive operations, who is not deployed as a working diver, and whose mission is to provide dive safety. He/she shall remain enlisted on the surface and shall always act at the direction of the team leader to support divers on the bottom. The safety diver may be employed as a working diver if each of the following conditions are met:

    a. 1st No-decompression dive to less than 30 metres.

    b. 2 ° The divers shall dive together in the same working area.

    c. 3rd The first diver, after a reconnaissance dive, determines that the work area is safe and free of hazards.

    d. 4th Maintenance work on ships and infrastructures.

23. Rebreather, recirculator or recycler: diving equipment that recovers the oxygen content of a diver's exhalation for reintroduction into the breathing circuit.

24. Contaminated water: water containing any chemical, biological, radiological or radioactive substance and presenting a risk to personnel exposed to it.

Diving modalities.

The Royal Decree 550/2020, dated 2 June 2022, defines a series of concepts which are copied verbatim from it in order to have a scope of the basic elements involved in this activity. For the purposes of this summary work, the diving modalities defined as officially accepted in Spain and defined in this decree are:

1. Recreational diving: is diving that may be for non-competitive sport, amusement, recreation, pastime or physical exercise.

2. Sport diving: is that the purpose of which is the exercise of a sporting activity at a competitive level or preparatory to it.

3. Professional diving: is that which is carried out for the exercise of an economic or business activity and which cannot be carried out under the protection of the other diving modalities.

4. Scientific diving: is that which has the purpose of carrying out studies or projects linked to a scientific research activity and is carried out exclusively for that purpose by means of a permit from the Public Administration competent for the research in question.

5. Diving for the extraction of living marine resources or extractive diving: is diving carried out for the harvesting or capture of living underwater resources for commercial purposes within the framework of a management plan granted by a Public Administration.

6. Military diving: diving performed by members of the Armed Forces, or personnel under their direction, for the fulfilment of military purposes or tasks assigned to them.

7. Diving for public service purposes: that which is carried out by Public Administration personnel, with the exception of military diving, for the fulfilment of these purposes. This type of diving includes that carried out by the State Security Forces and Bodies and bodies dependent on the Ministries and autonomous and local Administrations.

8. The types of diving are: autonomous, semi-autonomous, free diving in apnoea as well as the basic ones.

The decree regulates the depths to which people can dive according to their age. For this purpose it determines the minimum age for diving activities indicated in the decree as 18 years, except for recreational and sport diving which will be 8 years, but establishes maximum depths for each age: between 8 to 9 years of age the depth limit will be 6 metres, between 10 to 11 years of age the depth limit will be 12 metres, between 12 to 15 years of age the depth limit will be 21 metres, and between 16 to 18 years of age the depth limit will be 40 metres.

Safety standards for professional diving.

Hyperbaric chamber requirements.

For professional diving activities, in relation to the depths and decompression times of the operation, access to a hyperbaric chamber should be guaranteed for divers within a maximum of six hours when the professional diving activity has taken place at a depth of less than 10 metres and with a decompression time of less than 20 minutes, and within a maximum of two hours when the professional diving activity has taken place at a depth of 10 to 50 metres and with a decompression time of less than 20 minutes.

The hyperbaric chamber must be available at the same place where the professional diving is carried out, moreover, when work is carried out at depths of more than 50 metres or when dives with a decompression time of 20 minutes or more are planned, for its use the hyperbaric chamber must meet the safety standards required for its commercialisation by the applicable regulations and it must always be operated by qualified personnel.

Eligibility and exclusion criteria for diver examinations.

In order to be able to approve divers, whether they carry out professional, scientific or recreational activities, it is necessary to evaluate systems such as: circulatory, cardiopulmonary, respiratory, otorhinolaryngology, endocrine, digestive, gynaecological, urinary, locomotor, neurological, integumentary and visual. It is also necessary to evaluate the psychological and psychiatric level of the patient, given the feeling of isolation that he/she will have at many moments of his/her working or recreational life, being alone in a hostile environment.

In addition, a series of studies, clinical and laboratory tests are required for the estimation of the diver's needs. Among the types of tests will be:

- o Body Mass Index (BMI).
- o Simple otoscopy and Valsalva.
- o Anterior rhinoscopy.
- o Airway audiometry.
- o Impedanciometry.
- o Visual acuity.
- o Colour vision.
- o Cardiopulmonary auscultation.
- o Spirometry.
- o Blood pressure.
- o Ruffier or Step Harvard test.
- o Resting ECG.
- o Ergometry.
- o Musculoskeletal examination.
- o Neurological examination.
- o Psychological assessment.
- o Analytical.
- o Sickle cell screening.
- o Tuberculin test.
- o HIV.
- o Drug detection.

- o Pregnancy test.
- o X-ray of frontal and maxillary sinuses.
- o P-A and lateral chest X-ray.
- o X-ray of the scapular and pelvic girdle.
- o Knee X-ray.

Contraindications for diving.

Medication incompatible with diving according to ADCI.

According to the Association of Diving Contractors International (ADCI), there are some drugs which, if taken by patients, are a contraindication to diving. Among these are:

- o Amphetamines, designer drugs, marijuana, cocaine.
- o Natural and synthetic opioids.
- o Phosphodiesterase inhibitors.
- o Immunosuppressants.
- o All antidepressants except low doses of sertraline.
- o Antipsychotics.
- o Muscle relaxants.
- o All forms of insulin.
- o Oral hypoglycaemic agents.
- o Anticoagulants and platelet aggregation inhibitors.
- o Benzodiazepines, barbiturates, anxiolytics and hypnotics.
- o Nicotine patches, Varenicillin and bupropion.
- o Beta-blockers.

When patients have suffered a diving accident, the recovery period can range from simple pain that resolves within 24 hours, to a ruptured round window that can take up to 6 months to heal. Each injury and each patient will require individual assessment.

Bibliographical references.

1. Colodro, J. Assessment of psychological fitness for diving. Published: 15 May 2020. Cited: 13 October 2022. Retrieved from: https://www.pstys.cop.es/pdf/Evaluacion-aptitud-psicologica-Buceo.pdf

2. Desola, J. Scuba diving in childhood. Physiological considerations and suitability criteria. Apunts. Medicina de l'Esport. January 2006; 41(149), 34-38. Spain, Barcelona. 2006. Cited: 13 October 2022. Retrieved from: https://www.apunts.org/es-buceo-con-escafandra-autonoma-infancia--articulo-X0213371706889759

3. Ministry of Transport, Mobility and Urban Agenda. BOE. 6745. Real Decreto 550/2020, de 2 de junio, por el que se determinan las condiciones de seguridad de las actividades de buceo. Spain, Ministry of Transport, Mobility and Urban Agenda. Year of publication: 26 June 2020. Cited: 12 October 2022. Retrieved from: https://www.boe.es/eli/es/rd/2020/06/02/550

4. Romero, J. Causes of unfitness in aspiring divers and swimmers in the Eastern Region. EFDeportes.com, Digital Magazine. Buenos Aires, Year 19, Nº 191, April 2014. Cited: 13 October 2022. Retrieved from: https://efdeportes.com/efd191/causas-de-no-aptitud-en-aspirantes-a-buzos.htm

5. Juan F. González Rodríguez, Lic. Nancy Molina Gálvez, Technician Deisy Barthelemy Artze and Lic. María Elena Bolívar Murillo. Morphological evaluation and recommendation of norms for the Cuban diver. Cuba: Higher Institute of Military Medicine "Dr. Luis Díaz Soto". Centre of Aviation and Underwater Medicine. Rev Cub Med Mil v.26 n.2 Ciudad de la Habana. Year of publication: Jul-Dec 1997, Cited: 12 October 2022. Retrieved from: http://scielo.sld.cu/scielo.php?script=sci_arttext&pid=S0138-65571997000200003

6. University of Cadiz. Criteria for the assessment of diver competence. Spain: UCA: Cited: 12 October 2022. Retrieved from: https://av03-ext.uca.es/moodle/pluginfile.php/43418/mod_resource/content/1/10.2.%20Criterios%20de%20valoraci%C3%B3n%20de%20la%20aptitud%20para%20buceadores.pdf

Maritime accidents and pathologies caused by jellyfish.

Author: Hannah Diermissen Rodríguez
Email: hannahdiermissen@gmail.com

General information on jellyfish.

In the text Poisonous marine animals of the authors: Josep Mª Gili, Dacha Atienza, Verónica Fuentes, Santiago Nogué Xarau, I want to develop the topic about jellyfish, which as the reading indicates are present in the Mediterranean and Caribbean area. However, in the pacific zone it is also possible to find them in the pacific zone of Costa Rica.

Jellyfish are marine organisms that inhabit open waters near the Pacific coasts, the Caribbean Sea in Costa Rica, as well as in the Mediterranean area. For example, near the Spanish coasts where, as the reading indicates, it is possible to find five species of jellyfish, among the most common are Pelagia noctiluca, Chrysaora hysoscella, Rhizostoma pulmo, Carybdea marsupiales and Cotylorhiza tuberculata.

Among the main morphological characteristics of jellyfish is the fact that they have stinging cells with a diameter of 2 to 50 µm, which are called nematocysts, and which reach their maximum concentration in the tentacles where they can reach 105-106 cells/cm2. However, accidents occur most frequently on contact with them, generally near the coast when bathers are in the sea area, and contact with them can cause allergic reactions.

Clinical manifestations.

Contact with jellyfish tentacles causes both cutaneous and systemic lesions. Reactions may be local, with linear, multilinear or serpiginous distribution, with rashes persisting for days, weeks or months, in the form of erythema, oedema, petechiae, urticariform reactions (including papular urticaria), vesicles and local puritus with severe pain.

The literature indicates that the burning sensation like that caused by a cigarette is the first sensation at the moment of the sting, followed by rashes which may appear cyclically for several weeks afterwards, together with symptoms such as cramps, nausea or vomiting and acute pain in the areas of irritation.

The venom initially generates reactions that are more toxic than allergic, as the pain occurs immediately after the incidence. When the venom enters the bloodstream, systemic symptoms begin to appear, followed by the appearance of late reactions, which are mainly immunological, reactions that could lead to severe anaphylactic reactions.

Treatment.

When a bather has been stung by a jellyfish, it is necessary to carry out the following therapeutic actions according to Gili, Atienza, Fuentes, Nogué:

i. First get out of the water and try to remove visible tentacle remains from the skin, preferably with gloves or tweezers.

ii. Secondly, do not scratch or rub the area where you feel the intense pain or discomfort.

iii. Thirdly, wash the affected area with fresh water.

iv. Fourth, do not dry your skin with towels or use sand, as this may maximise skin erosion and allergic reaction.

v. Apply a solution of acetic acid (commercial vinegar) to prevent the nematocysts that have not yet triggered and thus reduce the virulence of the bite.

vi. Apply cold compresses as soon as possible for 5 to 15 minutes; however, avoid direct skin contact with water. Cold promotes denaturation of the toxin and prevents it from passing into the bloodstream.

vii. Attend a health centre for assessment by medical personnel to evaluate the use of steroids and antihistamines to treat the injury.

viii. In case of muscle pain, muscle relaxants and painkillers can be used, and the use of antibiotic therapy is indicated only in case a secondary infection is identified.

Another review by Vega, et al (2004) in their article Jellyfish stings: an update, available on the web addresses the issue and how the South American part of Chile can develop symptomatology and the management of this.

Bibliographical references.

1. Gili, et. al. (2022) POISONOUS MARINE ANIMALS. Species, location, manifestations in case of contact, sting or bite, treatment and prevention. Menarini Scientific Area. Revised: 10 October 2022. Available at: https://av03-ext.uca.es/moodle/mod/resource/view.php?id=29546

2. Vega, et al (2004). Jellyfish stings: an update. Revised: 10 October 2022. Available at: https://www.scielo.cl/pdf/rmc/v132n2/art14.pdf

CHAPTER VI. PATHOLOGIES, PRINCIPLES OF ACCIDENT MANAGEMENT, LIFEGUARDING AND FIRST AID IN AQUATIC ENVIRONMENTS

Tourism and water sports accidents.

Author: Hannah Diermissen Rodríguez
Email: hannahdiermissen@gmail.com

Aquatic activities constitute a risk in themselves, given that they are outside a traditional environment for human beings. When analysing the behaviour of patients and the rate of accidents related to the practice of sporting activities, mainly in childhood and adolescence, it is found that there are high levels of trauma and injuries due to accidents in aquatic environments worldwide and in the European Union for the purposes of this academic review.

The reading indicates that death by drowning is the second leading cause of injury-related mortality in children under 18 years of age. Water-based recreational settings have also been shown to be the most frequent setting for a wide range of other types of injuries in patients on holiday on European beaches, mostly in the Mediterranean region.

An important element identified by the study was that most of the injuries could have been avoided if clear expectations and specific safety recommendations had been established for the recreational activity carried out by the tourists who finally ended up becoming patients for the services provided, therefore the application of adequate prevention measures can help reduce injuries in children and adults and that is the first major contribution of the reading to the knowledge and management of pathologies due to sports or aquatic activities.

According to the World Health Organization (WHO, 2002), death by drowning is the second leading cause of injury-related death in children in Europe, and in children under 18 years of age, this accounts for 25% of injuries or accidents of people attending an EU country for recreation.

One element identified by McInnes in 2002 and Hargarten in 1991 is that locals have an advantage over tourists when it comes to holidaying and avoiding injuries in recreational areas, and why? Well, tourists tend to engage in more sports and unusual activities compared to locals, and are also unfamiliar with the natural and structural environment of their recreational area (beach, river, lake, estuary, etc.).

This is demonstrated by the 2006 Tapadinhas report which indicates that in the case of children who suffered water sports accidents during the holiday period in coastal areas, 72% of those who went diving in swimming pools and were not locals had a problem, which again shows that locals do indeed have advantages over foreigners when practising water sports in areas that are not familiar to them.

However, it is also important to analyse the case of the use of motorised training devices in order to correlate the number of accidents and injuries suffered by tourists in holiday areas in relation to locals, the report (Norman, 2008) indicates that jet ski users are injured at a frequency 8,This situation can be attributed to inexperience in operating such devices as indicated by the fact that the majority of collision victims had less than 20 hours of jet ski riding experience as indicated by White (1999) in 1999. Therefore, among recreational motorised devices, jet skis are the water recreational craft that generate the highest number of closed injuries and drowning as a cause of death in the European Union according to Branche (1997).

It is important for readers to bear in mind that motorised water sports carry a double risk (the percussive aquatic environment coupled with the risk of the speed of the machinery), according to Lunetta (Lunetta, 1998) Finland has the highest drowning rates in the European Union, with rates between 30 - 40% of all drowning accidents resulting from water traffic accidents.

However, all the situations described above can be prevented and many of these conditions of death can be solved with something as simple as abiding by the safety measures required of customers, tourists, bathers and ultimately patients. It is estimated that 85% of the deaths related to recreational boating could be prevented with only the proper use of life jackets at the individual level and training of boat drivers in on-board safety and nautical first aid, as indicated by Treser in his report (Treser, 1997).

Bibliographical references.

1.	Branche CM, Conn JM, Annest JL. Personal watercraft related injuries. A growing health concern. JAMA. 1997; 278: 663-5.

2.	Hargarten SW, Baker TD, Guptill K. Overseas fatalities of United States citizen travelers: an analysis of deaths related to international travel. Ann of Emergency Medicine. 1991; 20: 622-626.

3.	Lunetta P, Penttila A, Sama S. Water traffic accidents, drowning and alcohol in Finland, 1969-1995. Int J Epidemiol. 1998 Dec;27(6):1038-43.

4.	McInnes R, Williamson, LM, Morrison A. Unintentional injury during foreign travel: a review. Journal of travel medicine. 2002; 6: 297- 307.

5.	Norman N., Vincenten J. Protrecting children and youths in water recreation: Safety guidelines for services providers. Amsterdam: European Child Safety Alliance, Eurosafe; 2008.

6.	Tapadinhas, F. et al. Children submersion accidents in the East of Algarve. Child Health Magazine. 2002; 28(1):19 - 29.

7.	Treser C, Trusty M, Yang P. Personal flotation device usage: do educational efforts have an impact? Journal of Public Health Policy. 1997; 18(3): 346-56

8.	White MW; Cheatham ML. The underestimated impact of personal watercraft injuries. American Surgeon. 1999; 65(9): 865 - 9.

9.   World Health Organization. The Injury Chartbook: A graphical overview
       of the global burden of injuries. Geneva; 2002.

Pathologies in SAILING water sports.

Author: William Gutiérrez Sandí
Email: wgutierrezs@hotmail.com

Water activities are very attractive sports for the population, and the fact that we find ourselves practising sports in aquatic environments some involve low costs, without great complication, but others require special skills and may involve higher costs such as SAILING sports.

As Shephard (1990) points out, sailing sports are currently highly complex sports. There are currently hundreds of different boats, each with its own characteristics, as well as very different physical and technical demands, which can lead to people suffering from various types of injuries, but mainly of musculoskeletal origin.

The most common injuries in sailing are acute injuries, as in any other sport: wounds, abrasions, contusions against the equipment itself (boom, mast, etc.), burns, sprains, muscle and ligament tears, fractures, etc. However, the regular practice of these sports at a competitive level generates the appearance of another series of pathologies, but of a chronic type.

This is due to an overload of mechanical work in certain joints and muscle groups, which will have to do with the types of boat and the angles of attack and positioning of the athlete when performing the sporting gestures.

Each type of boat and each position on the boat implies specific patterns of injury mechanism, related to various factors as indicated by Ullis (1984):

i.   The position adopted during navigation should be assessed.

ii. Correlate the forces acting on the different apparatuses and systems of the body.

iii. Estimate the different physiological or energy demands of each type of vessel.

iv. The structure of the devices for sailing (SAILS, boards, etc.), which differ enormously from individual dinghy sailing (sailboards, laser, finn...), etc.

v.   Wind conditions play a predominant role in the physical and technical demands of sailing, and are also most implicated in the occurrence of injuries.

According to Schaefer (2000) and Allen (1999), winds of 17-20 knots and above cause most injuries.

It is possible to make a quick classification of injuries according to their mechanism of trauma, and which ones involve damage to the health of the athlete. Trauma injuries can be classified as follows:

i. Acute pathologies by direct mechanism such as, for example, incised-contuse injuries, contusions, muscle ruptures and bone fractures. There are also acute injuries by indirect mechanism such as ligament injuries (knee, ankle), muscle injuries (contractures, strains, fibrillar ruptures, etc.).

ii. Chronic injuries where it is possible to identify muscle injuries due to overloads with ruptures, lumbago, tendon injuries where it is possible to identify those corresponding to the rotator cuff, epicondyle/epicondyle, biceps femoris.

iii. Nerve injuries where there are lesions corresponding to median nerve compression syndrome or carpal tunnel syndrome, compression of the posterior branch of the nerve. Radial (Froehse's arcade).

iv. It is possible to find lesions corresponding to compartment syndromes in regions such as the forearms (flexor and extensor compartments) or in the region of the tibialis anterior muscle.

On the other hand, there are non-traumatological injuries that can also present acute or chronic pathologies in patients (the athlete) due to exposure to the environment and the conditions of the sport they practice. Among this type of injuries we can find:

i. ENT injuries such as ruptured eardrum and otitis externa.

ii. Skin lesions including sunburn, blisters on the palms of hands and feet.

iii. Eye injuries such as actinic conjunctivitis, retinal burn lesions, and the normal process of decreasing visual ability with age.

Finally, an important aspect to consider not only in water sports involving SAILING, but in general in any water sport activity or water rescue activity is what concerns the so-called fundamental rules in any form of water rescue (Scholne, 1994) which would encompass both water rescue and sea rescue and are just three basic principles:

First: caution: If you don't know, don't act.
Second: education: You never stop learning.
Third: prevention: Don't put off until tomorrow what you can do today.

This, together with basic components such as equipment preparation, sailor preparation and assessment of sailing conditions, makes the activity safer for all participants, and especially for you as an individual or as part of a crew.

Bibliographical references.

1. Allen JB. Sports medicine and sailing. *Phys Med Rehabil Clin N Am* 1999; 10:49-65.

2. Schaefer O. Injuries in dinghy-sailing - An Analysis of accidents among beginners. Sportverletz Sportschaden 2000 Mar; 14(1): 25-30

3. Scholne C. Injuries in sailing: risks and accidental injuries in sailing surveyed. NewsFlow 1994; 1:6-8.

4. Shephard RJ. The biology and medicine of sailing. *Sports Med* 1990; **9**:86-99

5. Ullis K.C., Anno K.: Injuries of competitive boardsailor. Physician Sports Med 12: 86-93, 1984.

First aid in wound management and bleeding.

Author: William Gutiérrez Sandí
Email: wgutierrezs@hotmail.com

Injury control in aquatic activities.

Injuries can occur on land or at sea. However, the management of these in an aquatic environment is more complex than a terrestrial environment, added to the fact that vessels do not always have people who are experts in adequate medical or pre-hospital care (Moya, 2019).

What is a wound?

It is the loss of skin continuity caused by trauma or a foreign object entering the body. It is possible to find several types of wounds as indicated by Ilerna (2022):

- **Excoriation: a** rough rubbing of the skin against a rough surface.
- **Cutting**: straight cut on the skin surface or deeper cut caused by sharp objects, regular edges.
- **Blunt**: caused by blunt or jagged objects with jagged, rough and/or torn edges,
- **Avulsions:** tearing, total or partial laceration of tissue caused by sharp objects such as cans, zinc sheets, etc.
- **Punctures:** small entry hole in the tissue with a trickle of blood, caused by objects such as ice picks, screwdrivers, etc.
- **Perforating:** Entrance wound with or without exit caused by a firearm.
- **Embedded objects:** There is a possibility that you may occasionally have to care for a person who has a foreign body embedded in their body.

What should a wound care process look like in an accident involving bleeding and in an aquatic/maritime environment?

In dealing with such incidents there are a number of actions that should be taken into consideration as mentioned by the Mayo Clinic (2020):

- Do not remove the embedded object.
- Uncover the wound and determine the severity of the wound.
- Activate the 9-1-1 emergency system if necessary.
- Treat it according to its classification.

- Control bleeding.
- Immobilise the object in place.
- Keep the affected person at rest.
- Prevent contamination by placing dressings on the wound. Do not use cotton wool.
- Apply a gauze bandage, triangular handkerchief.

Bleeding control.

Application of tourniquet.

A tourniquet is a device whose function is the strangulation of an injured limb to stop severe bleeding. A tourniquet is used in cases where the application of pressure on the wound or at the appropriate pressure point and elevation of the injured limb is unsuccessful. Pressure may not stop bleeding from a major artery in the thigh, the lower leg or bleeding from several arteries simultaneously as a result of traumatic amputation. Once the tourniquet is applied, the injured person needs to be permanently monitored (Doyle, 2008).

If a special tourniquet is not available, it is possible to improvise using soft, strong and flexible material such as gauze, bandage, articles of clothing or handkerchiefs, so as not to cause damage to the skin, making sure that the tourniquet is at least one inch wide when tightened.

Placement of the tourniquet.

Place the tourniquet around the injured limb above the wound at a distance of at least 15 centimetres - never place it directly over the wound or fracture.

For complete or partial amputation of a limb, place the tourniquet just above the wound or amputation. The tourniquet should be applied slightly above the elbow and above the knee when the bleeding is in the leg and/or forearm.

Tighten the tourniquet.

Tighten enough to stop bleeding or blood flow, before placing the tourniquet there is a pulse in the injured hand or foot, lack of pulse when applying the tourniquet is an indication that it is tight enough, the reduction of blood flow from the wound should be judicious, after tightening a tourniquet correctly the arterial bleeding stops, however, the bleeding of blood continues until the veins are devoid of blood as indicated by Gonzalez (2009).

Once the tourniquet is in place, check it frequently, as well as the bandages, to ensure that it is not loose and additional bleeding and acute haemorrhage occurs.

Bibliographical references.

1.   Doyle GS, Taillac PP. Tourniquets: a review of their current indications with proposals for their expanded use in the prehospital setting. Prehosp emerg emerg care [Internet]. 2008 [cited 2022 Aug 26];1(4):363-82. Available from: https://www.elsevier.es/es-revista-prehospital-emergency-care-edicion-espanola--44-articulo-los-torniquetes-una-revision-sus-13130845

2.   González Alonso V, Cuadra Madrid ME, Usero Pérez MC, Colmenar Jarillo G, Sánchez Gil MA. Control of external bleeding in combat. Prehosp emerg emerg care [Internet]. 2009 [cited 2022 Aug 26];2(4):293-304. Available from: https://www.elsevier.es/es-revista-prehospital-emergency-care-edicion-espanola--44-articulo-control-hemorragia-externa-combate-X1888402409460652

3.   Wounds: What types are there and how should you treat them? [Internet]. ILERNA Online blog. 2019 [cited 2022 Aug 26]. Available from: https://www.ilerna.es/blog/aprende-con-ilerna-online/sanidad/heridas-tipos-curas/

4.   Mora Jaime. Basic First Aid. San José, C R: INA, 2019; 03: 35-37

5.   Heavy bleeding: first aid [Internet]. Mayo Clinic. 2020 [cited 2022 Aug 26]. Available from: https://www.mayoclinic.org/es-es/first-aid/first-aid-severe-bleeding/basics/art-20056661

Fundamentals of water rescue.

Author: William Gutiérrez Sandí
Email: wgutierrezs@hotmail.com

Aquatic activities are a percé for the generation of different types of injuries. Traumatisms are among the most common injuries among people who practice musculoskeletal activities, as indicated by Allen (1999). In this section we will first review in a very general way the classification of the most common injuries and/or fractures proposed in aquatic activities and then the injuries related to musculoskeletal activities.

Bone structures and functions.

Bones are hard, whitish, tough organs and the skeleton is a collection of bones, of which there are 206 bones in total. The skeleton can be separated into axial and appendicular, into trunk where the spine, ribs and sternum are found.

Bones have a supporting function in the body (passive part of the musculoskeletal system), as well as a lever function due to the muscles that are inserted into the bones via tendons. They are also protectors of internal organs and carry out metabolic functions such as calcium and phosphorus metabolism and haematopoietic function thanks to the bone marrow.

Bone structure and physiology.

Composition of the bone tissue.

The bone composite is composed of:

- Bone cells:
    - Osteoblasts: young cells. anabolic function (bone formation).
    - Osteocytes: mature or adult cells. metabolic function (maintenance of bone already formed).
    - Osteoclasts: catabolic function (destruction of useless parts of the bone).
- Matrix or organic material: ostein, ossein or osteoid. composed of:
    - Collagen fibres provide strength to the bone, preventing it from becoming fragile.
    - A fundamental substance (mucopolysaccharides), it provides a medium for the deposition of mineral salts.
- Matrix or inorganic material: composed of mineral salts (calcium and phosphorus, which bind together to form calcium phosphate or hydroxyapatite), which are responsible for the hardness of the bone.

It can be segmented into two main segments:

- Periosteum: fibrous connective tissue membrane that externally surrounds the bone except at the articular surfaces. function: protection and thickening of the bone.

- Endosteum: inner periosteum. connective tissue membrane lining the medullary cavity.

Bone lesions.

Definition.

A bone lesion is defined as a lesion that causes a break in the continuity of the bone, i.e. a discontinuity in the periosteum.

Symptoms.

The symptomatology of fractures of different types is very varied. The main signs include functional impotence, swelling, pain, possible deformity, crepitus (crackling).

The patient with a bone injury (fracture) usually adopts an antalgic position. For example, if there is a trauma that has resulted in a fracture in the hip region, the patient will be seen lying down with the lower extremity in external rotation; another example is a fracture of the wrist (Colles), which is very common, especially in children.

When health care workers, whether out-of-hospital or in-hospital, are confronted with blunt trauma in older people (< 60 years), fractures should be suspected.

Classification of bone lesions.

Regarding the classification of fractures, Hernández, et al (2012) and the Mayo Clinic (2022) group them into:

a. Open.

b. Closed.

    i.   Simple.
    ii.   Displaced.
    iii. In comminute.
    iv. On green stem (children).
    v.   Capillary fissure or trace.
    vi. By uprooting.

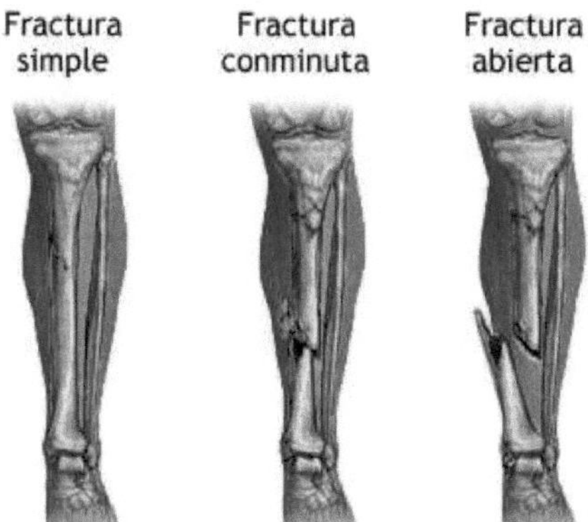

Figure 13. Bone fractures.
Source: https://sp.depositphotos.com/stock-photos/sistema-muscular.html

Treatment of bone injuries.

For their management, the mechanism of trauma and whether they are open or closed injuries must be known.

In the case of open injuries, the wound is superficially cleaned, attempts are made to stop bleeding, immobilisation is carried out, blood pressure is monitored and the patient is evacuated.

In the case of closed injuries, the patient is monitored for constants, immobilised, reassured (no painkillers or analgesics) and evacuated to hospital for radiographic diagnosis.

Spinal injuries.

Backbone structure.

The vertebral column is made up of bones called vertebrae (33 or 34). It is divided into 5 anatomical regions:

- Cervical: made up of seven vertebrae: atlas, axis, C3, C4, C5, C6 and C7.
- Dorsal or thoracic: 12 vertebrae. Thoracic arch: consists of a dorsal vertebra, a pair of ribs, the corresponding segment of the sternum and the costal cartilages.
- Lumbar: 5 vertebrae.
- Sacrum: 5 fused vertebrae forming the sacrum.
- Coccygeal: 4-5 fused vertebrae forming the coccyx.

Function of the spinal column.

The spine is a structure that withstands high-energy trauma, but this does not mean that it is not susceptible to injury. Its main functions include: head support, muscle insertion and rib attachment, spinal cord protection, haematopoietic (vertebral bodies).

Spinal (neck) injuries.

The spinal column is a series formation of cylindrical bones stacked one by one from the base of the skull to the coccyx (bone at the end of the spine). It includes the spinal cord which consists of long nerve conduits that link the brain to all organs and parts of the body and protects the spinal nerves. For Mora (2019) in some situations where cervical injury can be suspected are: precipitation, traffic accident, work accidents among others. About 20% of head injuries also present neck and spinal cord injury.

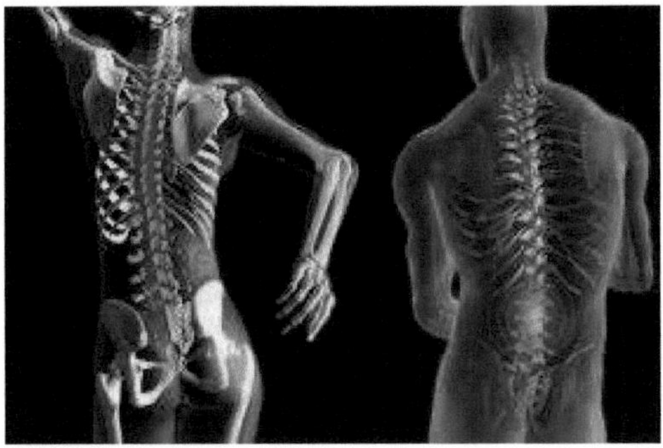

Figure 14. Structure of the spine
Source: https://sp.depositphotos.com/stock-photos/sistema-muscular.html

Signs and symptoms.

It is possible to find clinics presenting manifestations such as:

- Pain and functional impotence in the neck, upper and lower extremities.
- Tingling, weakness, burning and paralysis of the limbs.
- Loss of sphincter control.
- Deformity at neck level.
- Priapism.
- Loss of sensitivity.
- Nausea, vomiting and dizziness.

Muscular structures.

Myology.

- Muscle: organ whose main characteristic is that it has the property of contracting.
- Function: to execute all movements of the body (active element of the musculoskeletal system) and contribute to the maintenance of posture (muscle tone).
- Myology: part of anatomy that deals with the study of skeletal muscles.

Classification of muscles according to their shape.

- Fusiform or long: length predominates. Example: biceps and triceps brachii.
- Width: length and width predominate. Example: rectus abdominis muscles, latissimus dorsi.
- Short: no one dimension predominates. Intercostal muscles, orbicularis oris (around orifices).

Classification of muscles according to their function.

- Agonists or protagonists: They carry out a specific movement.
- Antagonists: Those who oppose the realisation of a certain movement.
- Synergists: those who collaborate in the realisation of a movement by helping the agonists.

Muscle sheaths.

- Epimysium or outer perimysium: surrounds the muscle as a whole.
- Perimysium (internal): surrounds the fascicles or bundles of muscle fibres.
- Endomysium: surrounds the muscle fibre.

Muscle classes.

- Skeletal: voluntarily contracting striated muscle tissue.
- Smooth: involuntarily contracting smooth muscle tissue.
- Cardiac, myocardial or myocardium: involuntarily contracting striated tissue.

Properties of skeletal muscles.

- Contractility: The ability to shorten in normal response to a nerve stimulus. It is the main property of muscle.
- Excitability: the ability to respond to stimuli.

- Elasticity: Ability to regain normal length and thickness after being lost due to an external mechanical cause.

- Tonicity or tone: A state of permanent tension of the muscles at rest, contributing to the maintenance of posture.

Frequent muscle injuries.

The various parts of the musculoskeletal system are subject to injury from a variety of causes. For basic care, immobilise the affected limb or extremity in the position it is in.

The Tear.

It is an injury consisting of ruptured muscle fibres or tendons, but without injury to the bone.

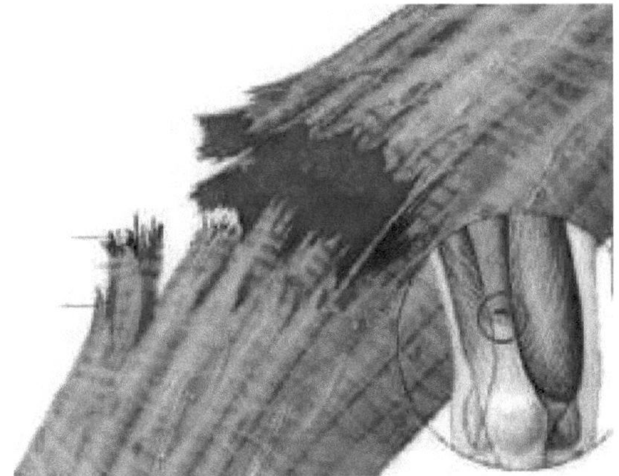

Figure 15. Muscle tear.
Source: https://sp.depositphotos.com/stock-photos/sistema-muscular.html

Sprains.

Violent strain of a joint that may be accompanied by the rupture of a ligament or muscle fibres.

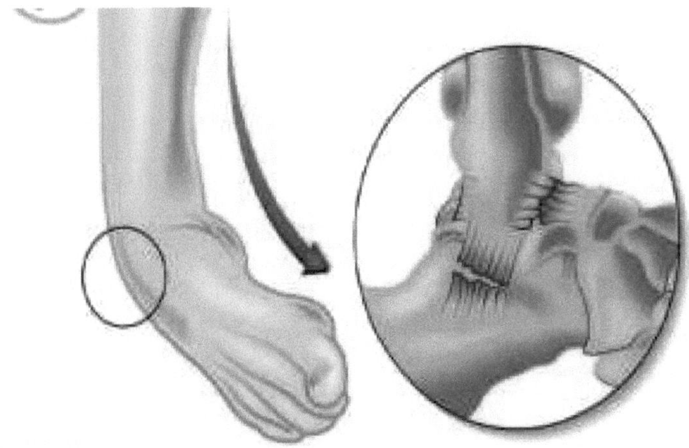

Figure 16. Muscle strain.
Source: https://sp.depositphotos.com/stock-photos/sistema-muscular.html

Dislocation.

It is the displacement of the end of a bone that is part of a joint.

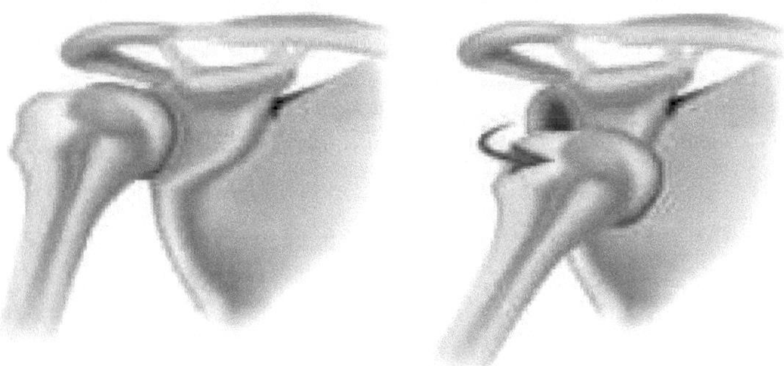

Figure 17. Shoulder dislocation.
Source: https://sp.depositphotos.com/stock-photos/sistema-muscular.html

An important aspect to consider in water sports and activities is that all participants may at some point require rescue manoeuvres and care in out-of-hospital settings with limited resources.

In general any water sport or water rescue activity is concerned with the so-called fundamental rules in any form of water rescue (Scholne, 1994) which would encompass both water rescue and sea rescue and are just three basic principles:

First: caution: If you don't know, don't act.
Second: education: You never stop learning.
Third: prevention: Don't put off until tomorrow what you can do today.

This is very important to be clear about in order to reduce the risk of becoming a victim of an aquatic incident.

Bibliographical references.

1. Allen JB. Sports medicine and sailing. *Phys Med Rehabil Clin N Am* 1999; 10:49-65.

2. Barcelona EP. 8 - PER - EMERGENCIES AT SEA - Escola Port - Aula Náutica [Internet]. Escola Port - Aula Náutica. Escola Port; 2015 [cited 26 Aug. 2022]. Available from: https://aulanautica.org/unit/8-emergencias-en-la-mar/

3. Fractures (broken bones) [Internet]. Mayo Clinic. 2022 [cited 2022 Aug 26, 2022]. Available from: https://www.mayoclinic.org/es-es/first-aid/first-aid-fractures/basics/art-20056641

4. Hernández EEH, Fonseca Monterubio A, Morales De Hernadez M, Elizondo Hernandez E. BP: Safety first aid. Bloomington, MN, United States of America: Palibrio; 2012.

5. Mora Jaime. Basic First Aid. San José, C R: INA, 2019; 03: 35-37.

6. Scholne C. Injuries in sailing: risks and accidental injuries in sailing surveyed. NewsFlow 1994; 1:6-8.

CHAPTER VII. MEDICAL CERTIFICATES FOR ACTIVITIES IN AQUATIC ENVIRONMENTS

Example Case I. Medical report for the issuance of a medical fitness certificate.

Author: William Gutiérrez Sandí
Email: wgutierrezs@hotmail.com

MEDICAL FITNESS ASSESSMENT REPORT.

The results of a case study of a patient whose personal data have been changed to protect his privacy, but whose medical conditions for the development of the medical fitness assessment for seafaring activities are maintained, are shown below.

Table 03. Format for patient identification for medical fitness examination.

DETAILS OF THE PRACTITIONER	
First and Last name: William Alonso Gutierrez Sandí	
Member No.: MED16970	Provincial Directorate: Puntarenas

WORKER'S DETAILS	
Name and Surname: José Alfonso Sacas Piedra	
Address: 200 m east of Liceo José	Location: Puntarenas
Province: Puntarenas	Occupation: Engine room chief, officer
Date of birth: 02/03/1978	DNI/NIE 6 0128 0875

DIAGNOSIS
Central Nervous System Pathology, G00-99 Nervous System Diseases, G43 Migraine. I10-15 Hypertension
Main diagnostic code: G43
Secondary diagnosis code: I10

MEDICAL-OCCUPATIONAL BACKGROUND
Family history: maternal grandfather: AHT, Sister: type II diabetes
Personal history: Patient presenting isolated episodes, but unable to perform work and/or personal activities with migraine episodes.
Vaccinations: Well vaccinated according to the Catalan calendar: last dose of hepatitis A+B.

Source: Prepared by Dr. Maria Luisa Canals (2022)

MEDICAL EXAMINATION.

- o Patient, male, 44 years old, qualified as a chief engineer. This is the third time he has undergone a medical examination, so it is a regular medical examination. The first, initial, was also carried out in Puntarenas, Costa Rica, despite the fact that his home and place of work would correspond to the provincial directorate of Santa Cruz, province of Guanacaste, Costa Rica.

- o Vital signs: Blood pressure: 126/67 mmHg, temperature: 36.3 °C, oxygen saturation, 99%, respiratory rate: 14 breaths per minute, heart rate: 83 beats per minute.

- o The two medical examinations were carried out in Panama, at the Einstein Clinic, with the same DUE equipment and equipment for the complementary tests (same conditions in the audiometry booth and of the personnel who carried it out, Mr. JI Ubieto). For this year 2022 the measurements are performed at the San Rafael Clinic in Puntarenas, Costa Rica. Therefore, the instrumentation base will not be the same to compare the evolution of the audiometries.

- o The first time she was seen in her initial examination by Dr. Alfonso Solís Guardia, a specialist in occupational medicine, who was performing his first substitution in Sanidad Marítima for Dr. Rimsky Sucre, the head doctor at the clinic. The second substitution by Dr. Sucre had indicated that the patient's basic pathologies were controlled hypertension, with Enalapril 20 mg orally every day, Amlodipine 5 mg orally every day, and for migraine he uses as a basic treatment: Omeoprazole 20 mg orally as a gastric protector, Ibuprofen 400 mg every day. For acute onset migraine, he uses Ergotamine 1 mg at the onset of symptoms, plus ibuprofen 400 mg orally, plus dimenhydrinate 50 mg orally, which can be repeated after 30 minutes if the acute symptoms are not resolved.

- o This third medical examination is of a preventive nature, after one year there are no new degenerative pathologies in relation to the patient's vision, hearing, respiratory and circulatory system. There is no explicit contradiction in the assessment of the restriction and the issuing of the ISM medical certificate.

- o The general examination is generally good, audiometry reports hearing of 20 dB for the right ear and 30 dB for the left ear, visual acuity (0.7 bilateral with Snellen optotype) which she corrects with glasses and/or contact lenses to 1.

- o As for complementary tests of the last examination. in the ECG, performed on 27.01.22 indicates: PR: 116 ms, QRS: 110 ms, QT/QTC: 386/405, HR: 79 bpm, with positive DI and positive AvF, for a normal axis.

o Spirometry FVC: 4.25 and FEV1: 3.70, and the patient is a non-smoker. It had not been performed previously in the evaluations at the other medical centre.

o Chest X-ray in normal parameters, performed on 27.01.22.

ORGAN AND/OR FUNCTIONAL LIMITATIONS.

o According to the Guide to the assessment of incapacity for work in PA - Chapter 9, ocular system, point 1.3.1 indicates that a visual acuity of 0.7 allows work with low to moderate requirements to be carried out. It requires visual aids and in this case with contact lenses and glasses corrects. The profession of bridge deckhand with lookouts requires a minimum vision in each eye. Visual acuity is an expression of the functional value of the retina. However, a visual acuity of 0.7 without correction can be a cause of unfitness. The RD 1696/2007 regulating medical examinations for sea embarkation - Annex 2, criterion point 2.7.1 in relation to the required visual acuity with or without correction is set at 0.7 and 0.5 in the eye with the best and worst acuity respectively.

o In chapter 10 on the otorhinolaryngological system it says that workers with exposure to harmful noise (80 DB) must be detected and preventive measures must be taken. In the case of mixed hearing loss, in which there is a transmission component and a perception component. The possibilities of recovery are only for the transmission component. Perceptual (sensorineural) hearing loss is generally considered irreversible. According to the INSS doctors' manual and applying the Klockhoff methodology modified by the Clinica del Laboro in Milan (2002) oriented towards the assessment of sequelae. In the case of our patient, he does not present any hearing pathology at this time, but the use of hearing protection mechanisms should be taken into consideration, given that he works as a manager in an engine room. Now, with regard to this point, the ILO-IMO/JMS 2011 and STCW 78/95/2010 Guidelines specify the hearing standards. Hearing ability should be at least 30 dB on average without correction in the better ear and 40 dB in the other ear, without correction in the other ear at frequencies 500, 1000, 2000 and 3000. This equates to speech distances of 3 metres and 2 metres respectively. This was no longer the case at her first medical examination, and as we can see, her hearing impairment has worsened as a result of exposure to noise at work.

o Regarding migraine, the Royal Decree of the BOE 313.31.12.2007 indicates ANNEX II, Criteria for the assessment of fitness for embarkation, 2.6 Diseases of the nervous system, does not classify them as a pathology that indicates a restriction for the issuance of the medical certificate.

o Regarding migraine, the Royal Decree of the BOE 313.31.12.2007 indicates ANNEX II, Criteria for the assessment of fitness for embarkation, 2.9. Diseases of the circulatory system. For the purpose of assessing fitness, the following criteria shall always be taken into account: family history of heart disease or sudden death, presence of symptoms and/or signs, functional capacity, location, prognosis, presence of electrocardiographic and/or echocardiographic abnormalities suggesting severe cardiac pathology even in the absence of symptoms, possibilities of treatment on board, risk of severe symptoms on board, risk factors and/or associated complications, therapy involving restrictions or limitations for the normal performance of their activities and specialist report. 2.9.1.7 Essential hypertension with significant organic repercussions or hypertension.

LABOUR REPORT.

o The organs of vision and hearing are not currently affected by any obvious occupational pathology for this seafarer who works as a chief engineer, with high exposure to noise and fluids that could have repercussions on respiratory pathology, at least for this survey.

o In the assessment of the initial examination according to the ILO-IMO/JMS 2011 Guidelines and in Spain the RD 1696/2007, they are usually stricter (but as these are minimum recommendations, it leaves the possibility for the medical risk assessment criteria to be adapted to the probable working conditions of the crew member and also the option to establish preventive restrictions).

o With regard to the guidelines for the conduct of medical examinations of seafarers, WCMS 2017, in Annex E. Criteria relating to physical fitness, with regard to common conditions, and in accordance with ICD-10 classification criteria, diagnostic codes, G00-99 Diseases of the nervous system, G43 Migraine (frequent attacks with disability), Likelihood of recurrences, disabling. For this the text indicates that there are three conditions:

  o Incompatible with the reliable performance of routine and emergency tasks in a Safe and effective manner. expected to be temporary (T), expected to be permanent (P).

  o Able to perform some but not all tasks or to work in some but not all waters (R). More frequent supervision is needed (L).

  o Able to perform all tasks anywhere in the world in the assigned section.

In the case of the present chief engineer, there is no record of having had any disabling events in the last 12 months and the acute events have been resolved in less than 24 hours.

o With regard to the guidelines for the conduct of medical examinations of seafarers, WCMS 2017, in Annex E. Criteria relating to physical fitness, with respect to common conditions, and in accordance with ICD-10 classification criteria, diagnostic codes, I00-99 Cardiovascular system, Hypertension Increased likelihood of ischaemic heart disease, eye and liver damage and stroke. Possibility of an acute hypertensive episode.

  o Incompatible with the reliable performance of routine and emergency tasks in a Safe and effective manner. expected to be temporary (T), expected to be permanent (P).

    - T - usually if systolic pressure >160 or diastolic pressure >100 mmHg until investigated and treated according to national or international guidelines for the management of hypertension.

    - P - with a systolic pressure >160 or diastolic pressure >100 mmHg persistent with or without treatment.

  o Able to perform some but not all tasks or to work in some but not all waters (R). More frequent supervision is needed (L).

    - L - if additional monitoring is necessary to ensure that the level remains within national guidelines.

  o Able to perform all tasks anywhere in the world in the assigned section.

    - If treated according to national guidelines and there are no disabling effects from the condition or medication.

Given that the patient presents stable BP values, with stable treatment for the last 36 months, with good adherence to treatment, with no acute episodes in the last months, this condition would not be a criterion for the non-issuance of the medical certificate.

o With reference to the STCW GUIDE FOR SEAWORKERS CONTAINS THE MANILA AMENDMENTS, 2010, issued by the INTERNATIONAL TRANSPORT WORKERS' FEDERATION (ITF), the patient meets the requirements set out for the position, therefore, the working conditions set out must be complied with by the employer in order not to harm the patient's health.

Table 04. STCW Seafarers' STCW Chief Engineer Profile.

Jefe de máquinas

NOMBRE DEL TÍTULO	REVALIDACIÓN	REGLA	
Título nacional de competencia y refrendo	Sí	I/2, II/1, II/3	T/E
Refrendo de reconocimiento del Estado de abanderamiento	Sí	I/10	R/E
Instrucción básica en seguridad - Técnicas de supervivencia personal - Prevención y lucha contra incendios - Conocimientos básicos de primeros auxilios - Seguridad personal y responsabilidades sociales	Obtenida durante los 5 años previos	VI/1	P/D
Cuidados médicos	No	VI/4	P/D
Embarcaciones de supervivencia y botes de rescate	Sí	VI/2	P/D
Técnicas avanzadas de lucha contra incendios	Sí	VI/3	P/D
Aptitud física	Sí	I/9	C/E
Familiarización básica en aspectos de seguridad	En la tarea asignada	VI/1	F/aB
Familiarización específica para el buque	En la tarea asignada	I/14	F/aB
Familiarización en aspectos de protección	En la tarea asignada	VI/6	F/aB

T/E Título exigido. C/E Certificado exigido. P/D Prueba documental. F/aB Formación a bordo. R/E Refrendo exigido.

Requisitos generales aplicables a la titulación de competencia de jefes de máquinas

Source: https://tituladosnauticopesqueros.files.wordpress.com/2017/02/stcw1.jpg

CLINICAL-LABOUR JUDGEMENT.

Based on the previous data and the STCW GUIDELINES FOR SEAFARERS CONTAINING THE MANILA AMENDMENTS, 2010, the guidelines for the conduct of medical examinations of seafarers, WCMS 2017, in Annex E. Criteria relating to physical fitness, with respect to common conditions, and in accordance with the classification criteria of ICD-10, the ILO-IMO/JMS 2011 Guidelines and in Spain the RD 1696/2007, the criteria established in the BOE 313.31.12.2007 indicates ANNEX II, Criteria for the assessment of fitness for embarkation, for the patient the pathologies that he presents at this moment are controlled, he has chronic medication that does not correspond to internationally regulated medicines.

If the employer is prevented, given that the patient has circulatory pathology which, if poorly controlled, can develop headaches that evolve into migraines or can generate angina or a coronary event if not properly attended to, that within the abortion kit and as part of the occupational health team, there should be an AED and medication for the management by TELECONSULTA of acute hypertensive pathology events while the patient can be taken to the nearest port.

Furthermore, given that he works as a machine operator, he should be provided with the appropriate protective equipment, so that he does not suffer hearing damage. In addition, he should have an annual check-up with an ophthalmologist to determine whether his eye pathology is evolving.

PROPOSAL.

The patient is given an APTO certificate and is advised to have an annual check-up with a cardiologist, ophthalmologist and audiometry test. The employer is instructed that the patient should not be alone when performing his work; however, this does not mean that he should duplicate the patient's function.

But do have other colleagues present in case of an acute migraine or cardiac event while working.

ANNEX III
MEDICAL CERTIFICATE OF FITNESS FOR EMBARKATION
MEDICAL EXAMINATION FOR SEA-SERVICE

As a result of the Medical Boarding Examination.

Mr/Ms: **José Alfonso Sacas Piedra** with DNI / NIE / Passport **6 0128 0875** has been declared *(the holder of this Seamens Book has passed his/her Medical Examination for sea-service with the result as follows).*

- _X_ **Suitable *(fit for sea-service).***
- Suitable with restrictions (*partially fit for sea-service*).
- *Unfit for sea-service.*

The term of this Acknowledgement expires on 08 February 2024.
(*The validity of this certificate expires the next*).

In Puntarenas, Costa Rica, at nineteen hours on the eighth day of February two thousand and twenty-two.

Seal of the Centre Signature of the Doctor Registration No.
(*Medical Center stamp*) (*William Alonso Gutiérrez Sandí*) (*MED 16970.*)
(Model Medical Certificate for the crew member overleaf)

Bibliographical references.

1. Guidelines for the conduct of medical examinations of seafarers. [Internet]. [Accessed 12 Feb 2022]. Available from https://www.ilo.org/wcmsp5/groups/public/---ed_dialogue/---sector/documents/normativeinstrument/wcms_174796.pdf

2. STCW Guide for Seafarers. ITGLWF. [Internet]. [Accessed 12 Feb 2022]. Available from https://www.itfglobal.org/es/reports-publications/guia-stcw-para-la-gente-de-mar

3. Royal Decree 1696/2007, of 14 December 2007, regulating medical examinations for maritime embarkation. [Internet]. [Accessed 12 Feb 2022]. Available at https://www.boe.es/eli/es/rd/2007/12/14/1696

4. Guidelines for the detection, diagnosis and treatment of Hypothyroidism in the Costa Rican Social Security Fund. [Internet]. [Accessed 12 Feb 2022]. Available at https://www.binasss.sa.cr/protocolos/protocolos.htm

5. MCA. Approved Doctor's Manual Seafarer Medical Examinations. January 2010. [Internet]. [Accessed 10 Feb 2022]. Available from https://av03-ext.uca.es/moodle/pluginfile.php/43195/mod_resource/intro/Guidelines%20MCA%2C%20UK.pdf

6. Revised Guidlines for conducting medical fitness examinations for seafarers. [Internet]. [Accessed 10 Feb 2022]. Available from https://av03-ext.uca.es/moodle/pluginfile.php/43195/mod_resource/intro/PEME%20Phillipines.pdf

Example case II. Review of the elements for the assessment of a case of a seafarer with musculoskeletal pathologies.

Author: William Gutiérrez Sandí
Email: wgutierrezs@hotmail.com

Application of the eight parameters for medical examinations in the musculoskeletal system.

In the following case study report on the functional assessment of these workers, an assessment of the musculoskeletal system is carried out. For this purpose, the 8-point assessment is carried out according to the international assessment guide for seafarers STWC.

1. Specific anamnesis.

2. Anatomo-functional examination in cardiology and angiology / or in psychiatry / or in the locomotor system.

3. Explorations: when, how, why and to whom. Scientific evidence for them. Age-specific screening if relevant.

4. Analytics: when, how, why and to whom. Scientific evidence for these. Age-specific examination if relevant.

5. Detection and monitoring of cardiovascular/ or psychiatric/ or musculoskeletal pathology of particular prevalence and/or morbidity and mortality or of interest in the maritime sector.

6. Specific assessment in relation to the pathology detected: time course, treatment, special checks, assessment of fitness.

7. Age-specific considerations.

8. Cardiovascular / or psychiatric / or musculoskeletal pathology clearly excludes: for work at sea or for certain types of work on board.

Content of the study.

1. Specific anamnesis.

- For the case study we will have a patient named María José Sirias Gabuardi, 32 years old, Costa Rican national, officer 3rd class in bridge.

- APP:

  - Hypothyroidism (diagnosed at age 10). Treatment: Levothyroxine 100 mcg daily by mouth.

- o Musculoskeletal injury to the shoulder. This case presents a medical assessment of a rotator cuff injury, of 14 months of evolution; injury which has been treated with pharmacological treatments, physical means, and physical therapy.

- AHF: DM2 mother, HT: father, Hypothyroidism: mother and sister.

- AUG: G: 01 P: 01 C: 00 A: 00.

- FUM: 05.02.22

- Planning method: dual oral contraceptive (oestrogen + progesterone)

- APnP: Smoking: refused, Alcohol: occasional, Illicit drugs: refused

- AQx: patient with no previous surgeries.

- Reason for enquiry: This is the second time for the renewal of your medical boarding certificate.

2. **Anatomo-functional examination in cardiology and angiology / or in psychiatry / or in the locomotor system.**

   Physical examination.

   - Anthropometric measurements:
     - o Chest: 104 cm.
     - o Left arm: 20 cm.
     - o Right arm: 21 cm.
     - o Waist: 76 cm.
     - o Gluteus: 109 cm.
     - o Left thigh: 55 cm.
     - o Right thigh: 54 cm.
     - o Right leg: 35 cm.
     - o Left leg: 34.5 cm.

   - Vital signs:
     - o Blood Pressure: 117/74 mmHg.
     - o Heart rate: 83 bpm.
     - o Respiratory rate: 14 rpm.
     - o Oxygen saturation: 99%.
     - o Temperature: 36.2 °C.
     - o Size: 164 cm.
     - o Weight: 69 kg.
     - o BMI: 25.64 kg/m2.

- Visual Acuity. Snell's test:

  o Right eye (without lenses): 20/20 OI: 1.

  o Left eye (without lenses): 20/20 OI: 1.

  o Binocular vision (without glasses): 20/20.

  o Ocular prosthesis or glasses: patient does not wear glasses.

- Chromatic Mink.

  o Ishihara films: no problems with colour recognition, colour blindness, Achromatopsia, Deuteranopia, Protanopia.

- Skin and mucous membranes: turgid skin, without lesions, spots, abrasions or allergies. Patient well hydrated, mucous membranes hydrated, patient without signs of dehydration.

- Ophthalmology:

  o Function of cranial nerves: PC III, PC IV, PC VI, preserved for eye movements.

  o Pupillary reflexes: direct photomotor, consensual photomotor preserved.

  o Fundus: no evidence of papilledema at the time of the patient's assessment.

- Otorhinolaryngology:

  o Hearing: no bilateral bone or sensorineural hearing loss, with right ear hearing 20 dB and left ear hearing 30 dB.

  o Pharynx and larynx: no evidence of infection, tonsillitis, pharyngeal erythema, candida. No morning sputum, or signs of altered salivation.

  o Mouth: with preserved teeth, no evidence of bruxism, with preserved bite, with shims on molar teeth, both in the upper and lower jaw.

- Cardiovascular: heart rhythmic, pulse regular, sinus, strong, with temporal, carotid, radial, popliteal, malleolar pulses present; heart sounds present, no murmurs, no return of cardiac cycle closure in systole and/or diastole.

- Respiratory: clear lung fields, audible vesicular murmur, no cramps, no wheezing, no hoarseness, no use of accessory muscles, no use of abdominal muscles for respiratory mechanics.

- Abdomen: soft, depressible, not painful on palpation, no evidence of palpable masses, no evidence of peritoneal irritation, no evidence of skin lesions in the abdominal region, abdominal pulse present, femoral pulse present.

- Neurological: cranial nerves: I, II, III, IV, V, VI, VI, VII, VIII, VIII, IX, X, XI, XII, with preserved motor and sensory function, with preserved deep and superficial sensitivity, with 5/5 strength in right upper limb, 5/5 strength in left upper limb, with 5/5 strength in right lower limb, 5/5 strength in left lower limb, with preserved eye-hand coordination tests, without ataxic gait or imbalance.

- Genitourinary: external genitalia according to sex and age, vagina normotensive, no discharge of infectious fluids, no bleeding, symmetrical external labia, perianal region with no evidence of skin lesions or visible skin sexually transmitted diseases. Normal micturition, no evidence of post micturition dribbling, no evidence of urinary incontinence.

- Locomotor: the musculoskeletal examination showed that the patient had preserved strength in all four limbs, strength 5/5 in the right upper limb, strength 5/5 in the left upper limb, strength 5/5 in the right lower limb, strength 5/5 in the left lower limb, no deformities in the fingers of the upper or lower limbs, no lesions or pathology of fungal origin in the cutaneous cuticle of her phalanges, no tattoos on her limbs. With preserved osteotendinous reflexes: nasopalpebral, masseteric, bicipital, tricipital, styloradial, ulnar, patellar, achilles, medial pubic (normal reflex: ++). With active movements in ranges of extension, flexion, adduction, abduction for left upper extremity, right lower extremity and left lower extremity. With pain on active mobilisation of the right shoulder on abduction for angles greater than 90°, for hyperflexion greater than 125°, with cramp on passive mobilisation. Pain on palpation in the region of the supraspinatus insertion in the shoulder girdle of the right upper limb.

Complementary tests.

- Electrocardiogram (ECG): the patient underwent a resting ECG on 17.01.2022 at 14:32 hours which reported: PR: 116 ms, QRS: 110 ms, QT/QTC: 386/405, HR: 79 bpm, with positive DI and positive AvF, for a normal axis.

- Spirometry: the patient underwent spirometry on 22.01.2022 at 09:46 hours which reported: FVC: 4.25 and FEV1: 3.70, the patient is a non-smoker. It had not been performed previously in the evaluations at the other medical centre.

- Chest X-ray AP: on 27.01.22 and which reports: in normal parameters.

- Audiometry: the patient underwent an audiometry test on 29.01.2022 which reports: patient who on general examination is generally good, in her audiometry she reports hearing of 20 dB for the right ear and 30 dB for the left ear.

- Fundus examination: performed on 29.01.2022 with no evidence of papilledema or intraocular hypertension.

- Snell assessment test at six metres: conducted on 29.01.2022.

    - Right eye (without lenses): 20/20 OI: 1.

    - Left eye (without lenses): 20/20 OI: 1.

    - Binocular vision (without glasses): 20/20.

    - No evidence of ocular injury or decrease in ocular injury at this time.

- Musculoskeletal ultrasound of the right shoulder: performed on 10.01.2022 with diagnostic impression: 1. Tendonitis of the long head of the biceps tendon, 2. Bursitis of the shoulder, reported by Dr. Ivan Sayago Masis, specialist in medical imaging and radiology.

- Laboratories. Conducted on 19.01.2022 reporting:

    - Haemogram: Red cells (RBC): 5.4 million/mcL, Haemoglobin: 15.7 g/dl, Haematocrit; 47.2%, Mean Corpuscular Volume (MCV) 87, WBC: 9.2 mil/mcL, neutrophils: 58%, lymphocytes: 34%, monocytes: 7%, eosinophils: 1%. Platelets: 196 mil/mcL.

    - Clinical chemistry: fasting glucose: 95 mg/dl, uric acid: 5.6 mg/dl, total cholesterol: 206 mg/dl, LDL cholesterol: 124 mg/dl, HDL cholesterol: 56 mg/dl, triglycerides: 145 mg/dl.

    - Renal function test: uraemic nitrogen: 14.3 mg/dl, creatinine: 1.15 mg/dl, estimated glomerular filtration rate MDR/CKD-EPI: 62.9 mL/min/1.73 m2.

    - Liver function tests: Total bilirubin: 1.2 mg/dl, direct bilirubin: 0.35 mg/dl, indirect bilirubin: 0.9 mg/dl, TGO/AST: 18.7 mg/dl, TGP/ALT: 17.0 mg/dl, alkaline phosphatase (ALP/FA): 148 IU/L, Lactate Dehydrogenase (LHD): 278 mmol/L.

    - Hormones: Human HGC (qualitative): Negative for pregnancy.

    - Hormones: TSH: 2.1 IUU/ml, Free T4: 1.1 IUU/ml.

3. **Explorations: when, how, why and to whom. Scientific evidence for these. Age-specific screening if relevant.**

   ALREADY answered in section 2 of this report.

4. **Analytics: when, how, why and to whom. Scientific evidence for these. Age-specific examination if relevant.**

   ALREADY answered in section 2 of this report. Patient in the age range of 18 to 50 years; therefore, there are no special age considerations for the issuance of the medical certificate. With regard to the underlying pathology of hypothyroidism, it is a pathology that is under control with more than 20 years of control by the patient.

5. **Specific assessment in relation to the pathology detected: temporal evolution, treatment, special controls.**

   - Time of evolution: 14 months.

   - Physical examination: on musculoskeletal examination, the patient showed preserved strength in all four limbs, strength 5/5 in the right upper limb, strength 5/5 in the left upper limb, strength 5/5 in the right lower limb, strength 5/5 in the left lower limb, no deformities in the fingers of the upper or lower limbs, no lesions or pathology of fungal origin in the skin cuticle of her phalanges, no tattoos on her limbs. With preserved osteotendinous reflexes: nasopalpebral, masseteric, bicipital, tricipital, styloradial, ulnar, patellar, achilles, medial pubic (normal reflex: ++). With active movements in ranges of extension, flexion, adduction, abduction for left upper extremity, right lower extremity and left lower extremity. With pain on active mobilisation of the right shoulder on abduction for angles greater than 90°, for hyperflexion greater than 125°, with cramp on passive mobilisation. Pain on palpation in the region of the supraspinatus insertion in the shoulder girdle of the right upper limb.

   - Musculoskeletal ultrasound of the right shoulder: performed on 10.01.2022 with diagnostic impression: 1. Tendonitis of the long head of the biceps tendon, 2. Bursitis of the shoulder, reported by Dr. Ivan Sayago Masis, specialist in medical imaging and radiology.

   - Treatment: Ibuprofen 400 mg c/8 hours orally for 10-day cycles, diclofenac 75 mg intramuscularly every 15-30 days according to acute symptoms before physical therapy.

   - Physical therapy: electrotherapy once a week in cycles of 10 sessions. These have been repeated for a total of 3 cycles of therapy. Dry needling, for nerve blockade with orthopaedic manual therapy techniques. Use of physical means with cryotherapy for cycles of 5 minutes with 4 repetitions in the evening or after work.

6. Assessment of aptitude for the performance of work activities.

The patient has two pathologies that may affect her work as a 3rd class officer on a merchant ship. These are assessed.

a. Hypothyroidism.

The patient has had chronic hypothyroidism for more than twenty years, with regulation of this pathology. With pharmacological treatment with Levothyroxine 100 mcg per day orally, with hormone test values every 6 - 12 months. With laboratory report of 19.01.2022, which indicates: Hormones: TSH: 2.1 uIU/ml, Free T4: 1.1 uIU/ml. Therefore, in agreement.

Based on Royal Decree 1696/2007, of 14 December 2007, Annex II, section 2.4. Endocrine, nutritional and metabolic diseases. For the purposes of assessing suitability, the following criteria should always be taken into account: presence of symptoms and/or signs, analytical data, possibilities of therapeutic compliance and/or follow-up, probability of severe symptoms appearing on board and specialist report, section 2.4.3 with regard to thyroid, parathyroid or adrenocortical pathology. Those patients with symptoms that prevent the normal performance of their duties on board or have inadequate analytical control despite treatment.

With reference to the Guidelines for the Conduct of Medical Fitness Examinations for Seafarers, Annex E. Fitness criteria for common medical conditions, under E00-90 Endocrine and metabolic, E00-90 is not listed separately. Other endocrine and metabolic disease (thyroid, adrenal gland including Addison's disease, pituitary, ovaries, testes). Likelihood of recurrence or complications.

- Incompatible with reliable performance of routine and emergency tasks in a safe and effective manner: 1. expected to be temporary (T): until treatment is established and stabilised without adverse effects, 2. expected to be permanent (P): if impairment persists, frequent adjustment of medication is necessary or there is an increased likelihood of serious complications.

- Fit to perform some but not all tasks or to work in some but not all waters (R) More frequent monitoring required (L): R, L - assessment on a case-by-case basis with specialist opinion if uncertain about prognosis or side effects of treatment. Need to consider the likelihood of disabling complications due to the condition or its treatment, including problems taking medication, and the consequences.

- Fit to perform all duties anywhere in the world in the assigned section: If the medication is stable, with no problems to be taken at sea and monitoring of the conditions is infrequent, there is no incapacity and the likelihood of complications is very low. Addison's disease: The risks will normally be such that an unrestricted certificate should not be issued.

Therefore, based on the thyroid hormone results obtained: TSH: 2.1 uIU/ml, Free T4: 1.1 uIU/ml, the fact of having 20 years of treatment, and remaining stable, would meet the condition of **Fit to perform all tasks anywhere in the world**, with the proviso that he maintains his medication in accordance with the prescription of his family doctor.

b. Musculoskeletal injury of the rotator cuff.

The patient has a pathology of musculoskeletal origin, based on Royal Decree 1696/2007, of 14 December 2007, in Annex II, section 2.13. Diseases of the musculoskeletal system and connective tissue. For the purposes of assessing aptitude, the following criteria shall always be taken into account: presence of symptoms and/or signs, prognosis, recurrence, functional repercussion on the performance of their duties, prior adaptation to the job, compatibility with work clothes and protective equipment, possibility of on-board treatment and specialist report. 2.13.1 Traumatic sequelae involving neurological impairment, ankylosis, stiffness, deformity or mutilation. 2.13.2 Congenital or acquired kyphosis or scoliosis causing marked symptomatology. 2.13.3 Degenerative, rheumatic, deposit or inflammatory arthropathies, refractory to treatment, with muscular, ligamentous or neurological involvement, with sequelae of ankylosis, stiffness, deformity or other complications. 2.13.4 Pathologies with: Loss of strength or muscle tone in extremities. Loss of grasping or gripping ability in one or both hands. 2.13.5 Joint prostheses. Exceptionally, those prostheses which, depending on the working conditions, do not compromise the average life of the prosthesis, shall be admitted with restrictions. 2.13.6 Herniated discs with neurological compromise. 2.13.7 Other congenital or acquired bone, ligament, tendon, cartilage or cartilage lesions that cause marked symptomatology.

With regard to the Guidelines for the Conduct of Medical Fitness Examinations for Seafarers, Annex C. Physical fitness requirements indicates the criteria to be taken into consideration and for which the patient could be refused a certificate. In the case of the patient there are NO RESTRICTIONS REGARDING endurance, flexibility, balance and coordination, size: adequate to enter restricted spaces, capacity for physical activity: heart and respiratory rates, and fitness to perform specific tasks involving the respiratory system. The patient also has no conditions related to high or low body mass/obesity, severely reduced muscle mass, musculoskeletal disease that makes it impossible to perform as a 3rd class officer, pain or limitation of movement, any ailment resulting from injury or surgery, lung disease, heart or blood vessel disease, and some neurological diseases. Although the patient has impairment to active mobilisation of the right shoulder, she has no functional limitation to safely and effectively perform routine and emergency tasks, tasks simulating routine and emergency tasks, assessment of cardiorespiratory reserve, including spirometer testing as obtained in the reported results.

With regard to the parameters assessed in Table B-I/9: Assessment of minimum physical fitness for ratings for ratings, located in Annex C of the Guidelines for the Conduct of Medical Fitness Examinations for Seafarers document, the patient reports for:

Tasks, functions, events or conditions on board: No problems with sense of balance, <u>with mild pain on mobilisation of the right shoulder when doing hyperextension or abduction activities with extended angles</u>, but no impediment to necessary movements and normal physical activities. The patient can, without assistance, climb up and down vertical ladders and stairs, negotiate high door thresholds, and operate door locking systems.

With regard to routine shipboard tasks involving the use of hand tools, movement of ship's stores, working at height, operating valves, performing a four-hour watch, working in confined spaces, responding to alarms, warnings and instructions, and verbal communication, the patient has no defined disability or diagnosed medical condition that reduces her ability to perform routine tasks essential to the safe operation of the ship. However, repetition of the same mechanical movement activity, extended hyperextension or abduction movements or excessive weight bearing may result in a functional limitation to the patient. However, under normal conditions the patient is able to: work with raised arms, but with limited range of motion with the right shoulder, stand and walk for a long period of time, enter restricted spaces.

Upon assessment of the emergency actions on board: evacuation, firefighting, and abandon ship, it was found that, although the patient suffers from a chronic rotator cuff injury, it does not constitute a definite disability or diagnosed illness that reduces her ability to perform emergency tasks essential to the safe operation of the ship, and that analgesia can correct her acute pain condition. The patient has the ability to: don a life jacket or immersion suit, crawl, feel for temperature differences, operate firefighting equipment, and use breathing apparatus (when required as part of her duties).

Therefore, the chronic pathology presented by the patient, who works as a 3rd grade deck officer responsible for deck activities, where she does not constantly perform mechanical repetitive actions that generate an exacerbation of her rotator cuff injury, does not constitute a pathology that makes it impossible or endangers her health condition to embark.

7. Age-specific considerations.

Patient in the age range of 18 to 50 years; therefore, there are no special age considerations for the issuance of the medical certificate.

8. Musculoskeletal pathology clearly excluding: for work at sea or for certain types of work on board.

This report presents a legal basis with regard to the Maritime Labour Convention, 2006, as amended (MLC, 2006): Inspections, Medical Examinations ... STCW 78/95/2010 Training / Authorisation centres, Issue of Specific Health Training Certificates Orden PRE/646/2004, de 5 de marzo (ES), Spain /European Directive: Order PRE/568/2009 of 5 March (ES), amending the content of the medicine cabinets to be carried on board ships as provided for in Royal Decree 258/1999, of 12 February / Annual aids, the resolution of 29/05/2013, of the Secretary of State for Social Security, which approves the action protocols for ISM vessels in the event of the need for mass evacuation of citizens, the Medical Records Database of Medical Examinations (SANIMAR, 1985) / Hospitalisation / Medical Consultations by Radio / CTM Certificates 2006 Vessel Inspection / Segumar (Fishing Inspections), of First Aid Kits, (FARMAR). It also complies with WHO/ILO/IMO International Guidelines 1997, ILO/IMO 2011, CTM 2006 and soon the fisheries, sets out the standard content of the Medical Certificate of Embarkation.

In addition, as developed in section six of this report in accordance with: Real Decreto 1696/2007, de 14 de diciembre 2007, en su anexo II, apartados, 2.4 y 2.13. con las Anexo E. Criteria relating to physical fitness with respect to common conditions, in section E00-90 Endocrine and metabolic and Annex C. Requirements for physical fitness, the occupational risk regulations of the National Insurance Institute (INS) and the regulations for the management of thyroid pathology of the CCSS in Costa Rica, the patient **has no absolute restrictions for the issuance of her medical boarding certificate**.

Bibliographical references

1. Guidelines for the conduct of medical examinations of seafarers. [Internet]. [Accessed 12 Feb 2022]. Available from https://www.ilo.org/wcmsp5/groups/public/---ed_dialogue/---sector/documents/normaliveinstrument/wcms_174796.pdf

2. STCW Guide for Seafarers. ITGLWF. [Internet]. [Accessed 12 Feb 2022]. Available from https://www.itfglobal.org/es/reports-publications/guia-stcw-para-la-gente-de-mar

3. Royal Decree 1696/2007, of 14 December 2007, regulating medical examinations for maritime embarkation. [Internet]. [Accessed 12 Feb 2022]. Available at https://www.boe.es/eli/es/rd/2007/12/14/1696

4. MCA. Approved Doctor's Manual Seafarer Medical Examinations. January 2010. [Internet]. [Accessed 10 Feb 2022]. Available from https://av03-ext.uca.es/moodle/pluginfile.php/43195/mod_resource/intro/Guidelines%20MCA%2C%20UK.pdf

5. Revised Guidlines for conducting medical fitness examinations for seafarers. [Internet]. [Accessed 10 Feb 2022]. Available from https://av03-ext.uca.es/moodle/pluginfile.php/43195/mod_resource/intro/PEME%20Phillipines.pdf

BIBLIOGRAPHICAL REFERENCES

1. African trypanosomiasis (sleeping sickness). Available at: www.who.int/mediacentre/factsheets/fs259/en

2. Allen JB. Sports medicine and sailing. *Phys Med Rehabil Clin N Am* 1999; 10:49-65.

3. Barcelona EP. 8 - PER - EMERGENCIES AT SEA - Escola Port - Aula Náutica [Internet]. Escola Port - Aula Náutica. Escola Port; 2015 [cited 26 Aug. 2022]. Available from: https://aulanautica.org/unit/8-emergencias-en-la-mar/

4. Bell R. Tropical Medicine. 4th ed. Leeds: Blackwell Science Ltd.; 1995.

5. Branche CM, Conn JM, Annest JL. Personal watercraft related injuries. A growing health concern. JAMA. 1997; 278: 663-5.

6. Canals, M. (2012). Maritime Medicine, a discipline anchored in the past, active in the present and with prospects for the future. El medico interactivo. [Accessed 21 Sep 2021]. Available at: https://elmedicointeractivo.com/medicina-maritima-disciplina-anclajes-pasado-activa-presente-y-perspectivas-futuro-20121017111138075445/

7. Colodro, J. Assessment of psychological fitness for diving. Published: 15 May 2020. Cited: 13 October 2022. Retrieved from: https://www.pstys.cop.es/pdf/Evaluacion-aptitud-psicologica-Buceo.pdf

8. Compilation of CESNI resolutions Meeting on 8 November 2018. ANNEXES. CESNI. [Internet]. [Accessed 10 Feb 2022]. Available from https://av03-ext.uca.es/moodle/pluginfile.php/43195/mod_resource/intro/Europe%20Inla nd%20Navigation%20Standards%20Medical%20Fitness%20Criteria%2020 18.pdf

9. International Labour Organisation Convention No. 113 (Medical Examination of Fishermen).

10. International Labour Organisation Convention No. 16 (Medical Examination of Young Persons).

11. International Labour Organisation Convention No. 73 (Medical Examination of Seafarers).

12. Desola, J. Scuba diving in childhood. Physiological considerations and suitability criteria. Apunts. Medicina de l'Esport. January 2006; 41(149), 34-38. Spain, Barcelona. 2006. Cited: 13 October 2022. Retrieved from: https://www.apunts.org/es-buceo-con-escafandra-autonoma-infancia--articulo-X0213371706889759

13. Digitisation, standardisation and globalisation of information. Case study on: Diabetes and Obesity in Seafarers. [Internet]. [Accessed 9 Feb 2022]. Available at https://av03-ext.uca.es/moodle/pluginfile.php/43196/mod_url/intro/Digitalisation%2C%20Obesity.pdf

14. Guidelines for the conduct of medical examinations of seafarers. [Internet]. [Accessed 9 Feb 2022]. Available from https://www.ilo.org/wcmsp5/groups/public/---ed_dialogue/---sector/documents/normativeinstrument/wcms_174796.pdf

15. Doyle GS, Taillac PP. Tourniquets: a review of their current indications with proposals for expanding their use in the prehospital setting. Prehosp emerg emerg care [Internet]. 2008 [cited 2022 Aug 26];1(4):363-82. Available from: https://www.elsevier.es/es-revista-prehospital-emergency-care-edicion-espanola--44-articulo-los-torniquetes-una-revision-sus-13130845

16. Infectious diseases of potential risk to the traveller. Available at: http://www.msc.es/profesionales/saludPublica/sanidadExterior/health/travelInter/cap5htm

17. Explanatory notice for the CESNI standards for medical fitness. CESNI. [Internet]. [Accessed 10 Feb 2022]. Available at https://av03-ext.uca.es/moodle/pluginfile.php/43195/mod_resource/intro/Explanations%20on%20Inland%20Navigation%20MF%20Standards.pdf

18. Fernández, A. (2012). Translation of the Textbook of Maritime Medicine - Manual of Maritime Medicine. Siri Pettersen Strandenes. Plataforma e-learnig FUECA-UCA . [Accessed 22 Sep 2021]. Available at: https://av02-ext.uca.es/moodle/course/view.php?id=4256

19. Yellow fever. Available at http://www.who.int/topics/yellow_fever/es/

20. Fractures (broken bones) [Internet]. Mayo Clinic. 2022 [cited 2022 Aug 26, 2022]. Available from: https://www.mayoclinic.org/es-es/first-aid/first-aid-fractures/basics/art-20056641.

21. GARRISON, H.: **History of Medicine**. Espasa-Calpe. Madrid, 1921.

22. Gili, et. al. (2022) POISONOUS MARINE ANIMALS. Species, location, manifestations in case of contact, sting or bite, treatment and prevention. Menarini Scientific Area. Revised: 10 October 2022. Available at: https://av03-ext.uca.es/moodle/mod/resource/view.php?id=29546

23. Goethe W. Manual of Nautical Medicine. ISM. Spriger-Verlag Ibérica. Barcelona, 1992.

24. González Alonso V, Cuadra Madrid ME, Usero Pérez MC, Colmenar Jarillo G, Sánchez Gil MA. Control of external bleeding in combat. Prehosp emerg emerg care [Internet]. 2009 [cited 2022 Aug 26];2(4):293-304. Available from: https://www.elsevier.es/es-revista-prehospital-emergency-care-edicion-espanola--44-articulo-control-hemorragia-externa-combate-X1888402409460652

25. Guanacaste at altitude. [Internet]. [Accessed 3 Feb 2022]. Available at https://www.guanacastealaaltura.com/index.php/el-pais/item/1411-ina-capacita-a-tripulantes-de-embarcaciones

26. International Medical Guide on Board. World Health Organization. Geneva, 1989.

27. Health Guide on board. Instituto Social de la Marina. Madrid, 2001.

28. STCW Guide for Seafarers. ITGLWF. [Internet]. [Accessed 12 Feb 2022]. Available from https://www.itfglobal.org/es/reports-publications/guia-stcw-para-la-gente-de-mar

29. Guidelines for the detection, diagnosis and treatment of Hypothyroidism in the Costa Rican Social Security Fund. [Internet]. [Accessed 12 Feb 2022]. Available at https://www.binasss.sa.cr/protocolos/protocolos.htm

30. GUIDELINES FOR APPROVED CLINICS The definitive standards for all approved clinics when part of the PEME programme. [Internet]. [Accessed 10 Feb 2022]. Available from https://av03-ext.uca.es/moodle/pluginfile.php/43195/mod_resource/intro/PEME%20Crui se%20Ships.pdf

31. Hargarten SW, Baker TD, Guptill K. Overseas fatalities of United States citizen travelers: an analysis of deaths related to international travel. Ann of Emergency Medicine. 1991; 20: 622-626.

32. Hernández EEH, Fonseca Monterubio A, Morales De Hernadez M, Elizondo Hernandez E. BP: Safety first aid. Bloomington, MN, United States of America: Palibrio; 2012.

33. IMO (2009). Conventions, International Maritime Organisation, London. [Accessed 22 Sep 2021]. Available at: https://www.imo.org/en/About/Conventions/Pages/ListOfConventions.aspx

34. National Learning Institute. [Internet]. [Accessed 3 Feb 2022]. Available from https://www.ina.ac.cr/Noticias/Lists/EntradasDeBlog/Post.aspx?ID=68

35. Law 31/1995 of 8 November 1995 on the Prevention of Occupational Risks.

36. Wounds: What types are there and how should you treat them? [Internet]. ILERNA Online blog. 2019 [cited 2022 Aug 26]. Available from: https://www.ilerna.es/blog/aprende-con-ilerna-online/sanidad/heridas-tipos-curas/

37. Law 14/1986 of 25 April 1986 on General Health.

38. Lunetta P, Penttila A, Sama S. Water traffic accidents, drowning and alcohol in Finland, 1969-1995. Int J Epidemiol. 1998 Dec;27(6):1038-43.

39. MCA. Approved Doctor's Manual Seafarer Medical Examinations. January 2010. [Internet]. [Accessed 10 Feb 2022]. Available from https://av03-ext.uca.es/moodle/pluginfile.php/43195/mod_resource/intro/Guidelines%20 MCA%2C%20UK.pdf

40. McInnes R, Williamson, LM, Morrison A. Unintentional injury during foreign travel: a review. Journal of travel medicine. 2002; 6 : 297- 307.

41. Occupational Medicine. Protocols and action practices. Vicente MªT, Ramírez MªV, Murcia JJ. Letrera Publicaciones S.L. Bilbao, 2.008.

42. Mestré, Fernando. Protocol to be applied in medical examinations for embarkation related to the manual handling of loads. Expert Programme in Maritime Health. UCA, Spain

43. Ministry of Transport, Mobility and Urban Agenda. BOE. 6745. Real Decreto 550/2020, de 2 de junio, por el que se determinan las condiciones de seguridad de las actividades de buceo. Spain, Ministry of Transport, Mobility and Urban Agenda. Year of publication: 26 June 2020. Cited: 12 October 2022. Retrieved from: https://www.boe.es/eli/es/rd/2020/06/02/550

44. Mora Jaime. Basic First Aid. San José, C R: INA, 2019; 03: 35-37   .

45. Norman N., Vincenten J. Protrecting children and youths in water recreation: Safety guidelines for services providers. Amsterdam: European Child Safety Alliance, Eurosafe; 2008.

46. IMO (2002). SOLAS: International Convention for the Safety of Life at Sea, 1974, and its 1988 Protocol: 2000 Amendments in force in January and July 2002. Revised: 1 July 2022. Available at: https://labordoc.ilo.org/discovery/fulldisplay/alma993679053402676/41ILO_I NST:41ILO_V2

47. IMO (2022). Frequently Asked Questions on the Maritime Labour Convention. Revised: 1 July 2022. Available at: https://www.ilo.org/global/standards/maritime-labour-convention-old/faq/WCMS_CON_TXT_ILS_MAR_FAQ_ES/lang--es/index.htm

48. Order of the Presidency of 1 March 1973.

49. Piniella, F. Seguridad del Transporte Marítimo, Cádiz, 2009.

50. President Figueres. [Internet]. [Accessed 3 Feb 2022]. Available at https://www.presidentefigueres.cr/

51. Specific Health Surveillance Protocols. Manual Handling of Loads. Ministry of Health and Consumer Affairs.

52. Royal Decree 1696/2007 of 14 December 2007, regulating medical examinations for maritime embarkation. [Internet]. [Accessed 12 Feb 2022]. Available at https://www.boe.es/eli/es/rd/2007/12/14/1696

53. Royal Decree 487/1.997 of 14 April 1997 on Minimum Health and Safety Provisions for the Manual Handling of Loads involving risks.

54. Revised Guidlines for conducting medical fitness examinations for seafarers. [Internet]. [Accessed 10 Feb 2022]. Available from https://av03-ext.uca.es/moodle/pluginfile.php/43195/mod_resource/intro/PEME%20Phillipines.pdf

55. Romero, J. Causes of unfitness in aspiring divers and swimmers in the Eastern Region. EFDeportes.com, Digital Magazine. Buenos Aires, Year 19, Nº 191, April 2014. Cited: 13 October 2022. Retrieved from: https://efdeportes.com/efd191/causas-de-no-aptitud-en-aspirantes-a-buzos.htm

56. Sánchez-Caro J, Abellán F. Telemedicina y protección de datos sanitarios (aspectos legales y éticos). Ed. Comares. Granada.

57. Heavy bleeding: first aid [Internet]. Mayo Clinic. 2020 [cited 2022 Aug 26]. Available from: https://www.mayoclinic.org/es-es/first-aid/first-aid-severe-bleeding/basics/art-20056661

58. SCHADEWALDT, H. and GOETHE, W.H.G.: The History of Nautical Medicine. In Goethe, W.H.G.; Watson, E. and Jones,E. (eds.): "Handbook of Nautical Medicine". Springer-Verlag. Berlin, 1984, pp.3-19.

59. Schaefer O. Injuries in dinghy-sailing - An Analysis of accidents among beginners. Sportverletz Sportschaden 2000 Mar; 14(1): 25-30

60. Scholne C. Injuries in sailing: risks and accidental injuries in sailing surveyed. NewsFlow 1994; 1:6-8.

61. Shephard RJ. The biology and medicine of sailing. *Sports Med* 1990; **9**:86-99

62. Stanberry B. Legal and ethical issues in European telemedicine. European Telemedicine 1999.

63. Tapadinhas, F. et al. Children submersion accidents in the East of Algarve. Child Health Magazine. 2002; 28(1):19 - 29.

64. Nautical fishing certificates. International legislation, national legislation and STCW guidance for seafarers. Contains the 2010 Manila amendments. [Accessed 22 Sep 2021]. Available at: https://tituladosnauticopesqueros.wordpress.com/2017/02/25/guia-stcw-para-la-gente-de-mar-contiene-las-enmiendas-de-manila-2010-stcw95-uno-

de-los-cuatro-pilares-del-regimen-regulatorio-internacional-del-transporte-maritimo-junto-con-otros-dos-convenios-omi/

65. Treser C, Trusty M, Yang P. Personal flotation device usage: do educational efforts have an impact? Journal of Public Health Policy. 1997; 18(3): 346-56

66. Juan F. González Rodríguez, Lic. Nancy Molina Gálvez, Technician Deisy Barthelemy Artze and Lic. María Elena Bolívar Murillo. Morphological evaluation and recommendation of norms for the Cuban diver. Cuba: Higher Institute of Military Medicine "Dr. Luis Díaz Soto". Centre of Aviation and Underwater Medicine. Rev Cub Med Mil v.26 n.2 Ciudad de la Habana. Year of publication: Jul-Dec 1997, Cited: 12 October 2022. Retrieved from: http://scielo.sld.cu/scielo.php?script=sci_arttext&pid=S0138-65571997000200003

67. Ullis K.C., Anno K.: Injuries of competitive boardsailor. Physician Sports Med 12: 86-93, 1984.

68. University of Cadiz. Criteria for the assessment of diver competence. Spain: UCA: Cited: 12 October 2022. Retrieved from: https://av03-ext.uca.es/moodle/pluginfile.php/43418/mod_resource/content/1/10.2.%20Criterios%20de%20valoraci%C3%B3n%20de%20la%20aptitud%20para%20buceadores.pdf

69. University of Cadiz. U2. Regulations. FUECA-UCA e-learning platform. [Accessed 22 Set 2021]. Available at: https://av02-ext.uca.es/moodle/course/view.php?id=4256

70. Vega, et al (2004). Jellyfish stings: an update. Revised: 10 October 2022. Available at: https://www.scielo.cl/pdf/rmc/v132n2/art14.pdf

71. White MW; Cheatham ML. The underestimated impact of personal watercraft injuries. American Surgeon. 1999; 65(9): 865 - 9.

72. Wootton R. Telemedicine: an introduction. European Telemedicine 1999

73. World Health Organization. The Injury Chartbook: A graphical overview of the global burden of injuries. Geneva; 2002.

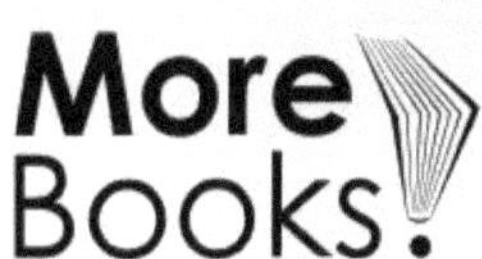

More
Books!

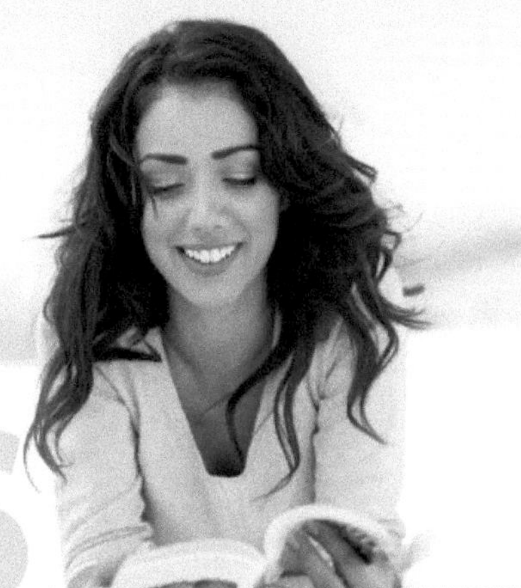

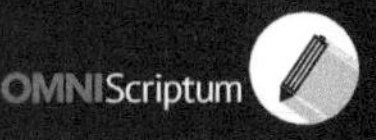

info@omniscriptum.com
www.omniscriptum.com
OMNIScriptum

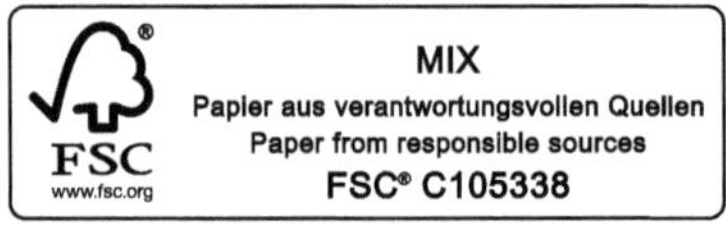

Printed by Books on Demand GmbH, Norderstedt / Germany